MADNESS

This book is an introduction to the uncertainties and incongruities about madness. It is aimed at all of those who are curious about this subject whether out of general inquisitiveness or because it is part of a formal course of study.

Using real case studies in order to explain, humanise, and bring to life the subject, Peter Morrall critically analyses how madness has been and is understood, or perhaps misunderstood. By contrasting past and present people who have been perceived as mad and/or perceive themselves as mad, Morrall presents core ideas about madness and critiques their would-be robustness in explaining the specific madness of the person in question, as well as their general relevance to madness overall.

Unlike many of its contemporaries, the book does not adhere to a perspective, but rather remains skeptical about the ideas of all who profess to understand madness, whether these emanate from sociology, psychology, psychotherapy, anthropology, 'anti' psychiatry, or the biological sciences of contemporary 'scientific-psychiatry'.

This book will inform and stimulate the thinking of the reader, and challenge those with preconceived ideas about madness.

Peter Morrall is an Associate Professor of Health Sociology at the University of Leeds, UK, who focuses on constructive critiques of the meaning of madness, madness and murder, and psychotherapy. He also rides motorbikes, sings, and plays the saxophone, but (so far) not all three at once.

MADNESS
Ideas About Insanity

Peter Morrall

Routledge
Taylor & Francis Group
LONDON AND NEW YORK

First published 2017
by Routledge
2 Park Square, Milton Park, Abingdon, Oxon OX14 4RN

and by Routledge
711 Third Avenue, New York, NY 10017

Routledge is an imprint of the Taylor & Francis Group, an informa business

British Library Cataloguing-in-Publication Data
A catalogue record for this book is available from the British
Library

Library of Congress Cataloging in Publication Data
Names: Morrall, Peter author.
Title: Madness : ideas about insanity / Peter Morrall.
Description: Milton Park, Abingdon, Oxon ; New York, NY :
Routledge, 2017.
Identifiers: LCCN 2016046394 | ISBN 9781138905511 (hbk) |
ISBN 9781138905528
(pbk) | ISBN 9781315695839 (ebk)
Subjects: LCSH: Mental illness--Case studies. | Mentally ill--Case
studies.
Classification: LCC RC465 .M68 2017 | DDC 616.89--dc23
LC record available at https://lccn.loc.gov/2016046394

ISBN: 978-1-138-90551-1 (hbk)
ISBN: 978-1-138-90552-8 (pbk)
ISBN: 978-1-315-69583-9 (ebk)

Typeset in Bembo
by HWA Text and Data Management, London

In memory of my mother Sheila Morrall
and friend Ray Graham
(neither *cuius erant copiose sanus*)

CONTENTS

ACKNOWLEDGEMENTS

Thank you to the editorial staff at Routledge, in particular Grace McInnes, Louisa Vahtrick, Carolina Antunes and Ed Needle for their support and patience, to colleagues and friends Pauline Philips, Gordon Teal, Karl Jarvis, Siobhan Hugh-Jones and Mike Hazelton, for their corrections and encouragements. Thank you also to the huge number of students from many different disciplines who have participated in my 'madness' courses over the last twenty years at Leeds University.

INTRODUCTION

They called me mad, and I called them mad, and damn them, they outvoted me.

Nathaniel Lee, 1684, quoted in Porter, 1987, p.3

Nathaniel Lee was a moderately well-known seventeenth-century playwright who became more well-known for the above pithy insight that madness may not be all it seems. The intention of this book is to present and scrutinise a selection of past and present ideas,[1] including those of the mad themselves, which purport to understand madness. The book is aimed at those for whom the subject of madness is part of a course of study, for example, in sociology, anthropology, psychology, psychotherapy, psychiatric/mental health nursing, general medical practice and psychiatry. It is also of relevance to anyone else who is curious about this subject.

The idea of madness held by Nathaniel Lee seems to be that what madness is and who is mad depends on the eye of the beholder. In his case, the beholders not only voted him mad but incarcerated him for five years in the London madhouse of 'Bedlam' (Porter, 1987). Here he was 'blistered'. Blistering consisted of shaving off the patient's head-hair and applying substances such as mustard powder to inflame the skin in an attempt to re-balance his 'humors'. Humors are the bodily fluids thought by the Ancient Greeks to be responsible for four modes of temperament: miserableness (melancholic), irritability (choleric), peaceable (phlegmatic), and optimistic (sanguine). What his physician, Edward Tyson, hoped was that Lee's madness would be drawn out of him through the pus which formed when the blisters became infected. Eventually discharged from Bedlam he was to die at the age of 43 years having been run over by a coach after falling over in the street while drunk (Arnold, 2008).

As early as the eighth century in the Islamic world, there were institutions which accepted the insane. These were elementary hospitals called 'maristans' and were first founded in the Persian city of Gundeshapur (Forcen, 2013). Bedlam was Christian Europe's first institution for the insane, originating in 1247 as a priory although it was many decades before it began to be used as a place of residence for the mad (Andrews, *et al.*, 1997). Over the centuries it was to change sites and names numerous times. It was to eventually settle at Beckenham in south-east London with the name of Bethlem Royal Hospital and is part of a large National Health Service trust. Moreover, its reputation has altered from one of infamy to fame. Whereas once it was associated with crude containment and dubious treatments it is today part of a group of internationally respected psychiatric establishments associated with sophisticated scientific endeavour such as the Institute of Psychiatry, Psychology and Neuroscience at King's College London (King's College London, 2016).

Virtually all institutions such as Bedlam (and in the UK, virtually every town had at least one, some of which contained thousands of patients), have closed down. Despite the demise of the large madhouses, asylums, and mental hospitals and dispersal of the huge number or people they contained, many more people are being 'voted' mad today compared with the time of Nathaniel Lee. But on what basis is the decision to describe someone or oneself as mad made? From where do the ideas originate to support such a description? How do understandings about madness affect its administration, how it is regarded and who does and who doesn't get designated mad? Is there a generally accepted comprehension of madness which goes beyond that of the eye of the beholder? These are the key questions tackled in this book.

Humoral Theory, and the concomitant notion of expunging morbid fluids through suppurating sores is no longer indulged by the medical profession. However, far from being understood better than at the time of Nathaniel Lee, madness has become a highly contentious area of academic study and professional practice. Over the ensuing centuries there have been, and still are, a plethora of competing explanations for madness, what it is and thereby how it should be managed – if it should be managed at all.

The vehicle for exploring notions of madness I am using in this book is a series of personal stories from different epochs and different countries as told by those who regard themselves and/or are regarded by others as mad. Ideas arising from diverse disciplines, including psychiatry, neurology, psychology, anthropology and sociology are applied to the stories. The credibility of each of the ideas is reviewed. In each chapter at least three ideas from a selection of these disciplines are utilised.

Some of the exponents of the ideas have specifically addressed the chapter's story while others have been chosen because they, I submit, offer noteworthy illumination. However, the individual whose story is being told is also offering an idea. The autobiographical basis of such stories is either explicitly or implicitly a submission of an idea about madness (Peterson, 1982). Both the personal and professional versions are presented as possible ways of thinking about madness (or at least the madness of the particular person in question). That is, the postulations of academics and practitioners as well as the narratives of the mad provide insights into madness. Some of the ideas overlap considerably, and they and their proponents make appearances in several chapters. As with ideas, only a tiny proportion of possible stories can be told in one book.

Imprecision and disputation

As indicated above, there is no shortage of viewpoints about madness, but, there is no one position which is uncontroversial and irrefutable. Each and every idea about madness is contestable. The divisions between madness, badness, and normality are blurred. There isn't even a generally established term for what I am referring to here as 'madness', or any one definition that is agreed universally. The 2007 Mental Health Act for England and Wales employs a teleological definition. That is, it is circular as it explains mental disorder as disordered mentality (i.e. disorder of the mind) hence does not afford clarity. Furthermore, it furnishes additional obfuscation by paralleling disorder with disability without any accompanying elucidation:

> '[M]ental disorder' means any disorder or disability of the mind; and 'mentally disordered' shall be construed accordingly.
>
> *Mental Health Act, 2007, Chapter 1, p.1*

The World Health Organisation provides a definition of 'mental health', and, because WHO is the most prominent supra-national health organisation, this is frequently quoted in academic and clinical literature and has been distributed across the globe as a universal health policy standard (Morrall and Hazeleton, 2004). However, it is imprecise and idealistic:

> Mental health is defined as a state of well-being in which every individual realizes his or her own potential, can cope with the normal stresses of life, can work productively and fruitfully, and is able to make a contribution to her or his community.
>
> *WHO, 2014a*

This definition of mental health implies that anyone who has not reached his/her full potential, coping with the normal stresses of life, working productively and fruitfully, and making a contribution to his/her community, is mentally unhealthy. Far from most of the world's population realising its 'full potential', there is much evidence of incapacity.

The WHO (2014a) itself records an increasing amount of mental disorder in the world. Thus an increasing number of people are not achieving a state anywhere approaching psychological fulfilment. Mental disorder has in the twenty-first century, according to the WHO, become one of the most serious groups of global health problems alongside cancer and heart disease. One in four people will be diagnosed with a mental disorder at some point in their lives. A fifth of the world's children and adolescents have difficulties with their mental health, and over three-quarters of a million people each year commit suicide.

Furthermore, certain social situations can impede severely the achievement and maintenance of optimal psychological contentment or even a less utopian state of well-being than that aimed for by the WHO. Amongst the dozens of global issues listed by the United Nations are the major obstacles to individuals realising their full potential: climate change, terrorism, AIDS, lack of food, water pollution and scarcity, population growth and terrorism (United Nations, 2015).

For one billion of the world's population living in dire material poverty is their state of being (World Bank, 2015). Violence remains unresolved as a serious social and moral problem globally. Ninety-million people live in conditions that run a high risk of degenerating into genocide or politicide (Wilkinson, 2005). Half-a-million intentional homicides take place globally per annum, but this is considered a gross under-estimation of actual illegal deaths as a result of interpersonal and State violence which is unrecorded (UNODC, 2014). A rise in social discontent across the globe is associated with economic, migratory, and political turbulence (Theodossopoulos and Kirtsoglo, 2010; Briggs, 2012; Lexington, 2014; Vanbergen, 2017). Moreover, there is no consensus amongst academics and practitioners about where the root of madness can be located. Identifying causation has consequences for how the mad should be cared for, what treatments should be offered, and whether or not there is the likelihood of a cure.

Social scientists mostly emphasise that madness and similar terms have been and still are utilised in the few remaining traditional cultures associated with the gods or God, the devil or loosely with nature and nurture, rather than primarily with personal biological and psychological pathology (Porter, 1987; Hirst and Woolley, 1982). Madness in this sense is a pre-medicalisation or non-medicalised signing of irregular and undesirable acts, beliefs and feelings. But the disassociation of madness from medical classification by social scientists does not necessarily if ever coincide with the provision of a resolute and indisputable substitute.

Disagreement over causation, however, has its root in epistemological as well as clinical predisposition. For example, medically trained personnel are likely to focus on 'faults' in the individual especially biological deficiencies affecting the brain, which could be corrected through physical methods of treatment such as drugs, surgery and electro-convulsive-therapy. Those who have been trained in psychology are also likely to focus on 'faults' in the individual's mind which could be corrected through psychotherapy. Those with sociological backgrounds are likely to focus on the 'faults' in society and thereby on social change as a remedy for madness. However, there are academics and clinicians who mix their ideas. For example, natural scientific and social scientific[2] ideas may be combined in an attempt to provide a less partisan and thereby a more robust exposition on causation. This then may lead to a combination of treatments such as a talking therapy with one or more pharmaceutical products.

Definitional accuracy let alone exactitude in comprehension is exacerbated because some notions about the nature of madness construe it not as an 'it' but as multiple 'its' or appear to mix-up the two. That is, there has been no consistency in the medical or social science literature over what particular states of human performance 'madness' embraces. Sometimes the medicalised states of schizophrenia, manic-depression and depression are implicated but at other times it is used indiscriminately (Burton, 2009). It may be presented as equating loosely to some, many, or even all of the alleged mental disorders which appear in the extensive inventories of the World Health Organisation (that is, its International Classification of Diseases – Mental and Behavioural Disorders: ICD) and American Psychiatric Association (that is, its Diagnostic and Statistical Manual of Mental Disorders: DSM).

Attempting to pinpoint which mental disorder or disorders from the hundreds of different types listed in these systems of classification equates to madness is problematic for two reasons: first, these inventories change over time (jointly there have been 15 versions to-date); second, they are essentially the creation of one region of the world (the West) and of one discipline (the profession of medicine) and thereby tend to downplay manifestations from others cultures and ideas from other schools of thought. Furthermore, 'madness' was used by medical practitioners who dealt with matters of the mind before the forming of psychiatry (for example, Battye, 1758) and still is by those who followed (for example, Wing, 1978; McLaren, 2007).

An absence of uniformity in what is meant by madness either as a portion of human performance or a term, and what is meant by mental disorder generally or any particular disorder, may be inevitable because what is considered normal and what is considered abnormal changes or isn't clear and consistent within social science as well psychiatry (Clinard and Meire, 2016). An intellectual allowance should also be made for the possibility of madness being something different to those ideas which so far have attempted to describe it. Could it be that no past, present or future idea is capable of fathoming insanity because it cannot be understood?

Acceptable terminology

The issue of definition brings forward a related contention, that of terminological acceptability. Two controversial terms, madness and insanity, have already been used. However, these (and other idioms such as lunacy as well as idiocy and imbecility when referring to what is presently tagged as 'learning disability'), were once considered socially suitable and entered into legal statutes and clinical text books. The terms idiocy and imbecility existed in legislation in countries such as the UK and Australia until well into the twentieth century. The term 'lunacy' was used until towards the end of the twentieth century in some countries, for example, India, which had adopted the language of their previous colonisers (Narayan and Shikha, 2013). 'Insanity' is derived from the Latin 'in' meaning 'not' and *'sanus'* meaning healthy with the mind later implicated specifically (Onions, 1966). This term can still be found in the mental health and criminal legislation of developing countries such as Botswana and developed countries such as the UK and the USA (Nsereko, 2011; Kimonis, 2015). The sociologist Andrew Scull (2015) admits that the term 'madness' is regarded by many as politically incorrect but until the nineteenth century it was the usual ascription employed by both the public and the would-be healers of people deemed to be psychologically troubled and troubling. For Scull, it remains a common-sense designation and one which is decoupled from medicalisation.

Reacting against the dominance of psychiatry, as well as the prejudice of the press and the public, some academics and practitioners adopt phrases intended to promote de-medicalisation and de-stigmatisation. The 'Time to Change' (2008) campaign by British mental health charities MIND and Rethink Mental Illness, and supported by a cross-party selection of politicians, commenced in 2007. It adopts the slogan 'Mind your Language' and recommends the expression 'mental health problem' instead of 'mental disorder/illness' as well as 'service users' rather than 'patients'. However, this does not wholly detract from medicalisation as it preserves an illusion to a medical condition by referring to 'health' and 'problem'. Others want to abandon any mention of health, ill-health, illness or disorder and diagnostic tags and refer only to personal issues, difficulties or problems. For example, radical psychologists foster phrases such as 'complaint-orientated approach' and 'psychological formulation' to replace systems of psychiatric diagnosis (Bentall, 2003; Johnstone and Dallos, 2006). These terms infer the epistemological stance of their propagators. Furthermore, it remains questionable as to whether or not any change in language will remove stigma given that for centuries the mad have been and continue to be defamed, no matter what jargon is favoured. It is also disputable whether medical appellations or any other argot, increase or decrease stigma (Ruscio, 2004; Morrall, 2016).

Given these shortfalls and discrepancies, I do not propose a firm definition of madness in this Introduction. Indeed, it would be contradictory so to do as this could confer compliance to one idea or another prior to their unpacking to test whether or not such conferment is deserved. In the main when commenting on the perceptions of psychiatry the rubric 'mental disorder' (or mental illness) or the name of the specific disorder will be made use of, but this should not be taken as an acceptance by me of medical definitional legitimacy unless stipulated as such. Otherwise, the appellation 'madness' will be used or, to avoid literary tedium, 'insanity'.

Power of psychiatry

Notwithstanding epistemological and terminological controversy, increasingly more mental disorder is being uncovered, increasingly more mental disorders conceived, increasing causative faults identified and increasing remedies invented by psychiatry. In Western countries, the psychiatric standpoint has dominated ideas for centuries and is now being transported throughout the world. The advance of and advances in psychiatry lead Allan Tasman, editor of the journal *Psychiatric Times* (which claims to be the most widely read publication for psychiatrists in the USA), to proclaim:

> We live in what is arguably the most exciting time in the history of psychiatry.
>
> *Tasman, 2014*

Whether or not such occupational excitement is warranted is debatable.

Psychiatry, because it is the prevailing perspective in the West if not the world (Mills, 2014), is given much attention in this book. The last chapter of the book focuses on psychiatry, and its propositions and practices are encountered throughout.

Since the profession of medicine took over the management of madness in the nineteenth century and fashioned psychiatry as a medical speciality other disciplines such as psychology, psychotherapy, social work and sociology have challenged regularly its dominance and continue so to do. However, psychiatry's epistemology is not a uniformly compiled or unvaryingly conveyed schema (nor is this so for any other discipline). There have been and remain striking splits within psychiatry regarding what exactly should be its *modus operandi*. For example, there are internal disputations over: whether genes, bio-chemicals, or pathogens trigger the major mental disorder of schizophrenia, and over the precise gene, bio-chemical or pathogen; the potency or not of the placebo effect for many psychiatric drugs, and the choice and effectiveness of medication for treating depression, anxiety and dementia; the validity and reliability of the diagnostic guidebooks. Moreover, there are psychiatrists who eschew some or much of the 'hard' scientific principles and procedures of the majority of their colleagues, preferring to concentrate on the 'soft' science of psychotherapeutic and social discernments and praxes.

Some European and North American psychiatrists in the 1960s turned on their orthodox colleagues and formed highly antagonistic factions. Moreover, unlike the rest of the profession of medicine in its relationship with its clientele,[3] psychiatry regularly entails overt and at times dramatic coercion. Some (ex) patients, hardly surprisingly, have objected to enforced treatment as well as what they consider to be the inhumane and disempowering aspects of their dealings with psychiatry. The idea of these self-described 'psychiatric-survivors' is to reveal the alleged abusive creeds and customs of the orthodox psychiatric system, and they campaign directly against the practitioners who are supposed to be or have been trying to help them survive madness. If you suffer from a physical illness (whether influenza, cancer, diabetes, or gonorrhoea) you would not expect, at any point in your dealings with your medical practitioner, to be potentially or actually compulsorily medicated, restrained, secluded or given electric shocks. If you suffer from mental disorder there are (mental health) laws which allow the psychiatric team (psychiatrists and other practitioners) to implement physical force to detain and administer treatments.

However, this book illustrates the uncertainties and incongruities surrounding madness not only concerning psychiatry but within the narratives of the mad themselves and within the theories of those disciplines who propose alternative interpretations and solutions to medicalisation. That is, although this book is written by a sociologist it is not (yet another) thesis *against* psychiatry. Nor is it indiscriminately *for* alternative (for example, sociological) explanations. I recognise that psychiatry has progressed and even if at times not progressive as a social institution some of its members have promulgated social and humane reform. The Bedlam physician Edward Tyson did vote Nathaniel Lee mad and was a blistering enthusiast but he also advocated hygienic and nutritious care and supplied money and clothing as well as installing out-patient facilities for his discharged patients (Arnold, 2008). From the outset of preparing to write this book *all* ideas – including the narratives of the mad – were regarded by me as susceptible to sceptical (but not cynical) disassembly.

Stories and ideas

Let me now present the people whose stories are to be told together with the main proponents of the applied ideas:

Chapter 1

Pierre Rivière was a poor French peasant who in 1835 used an agricultural implement to slay his pregnant mother, his brother and his sister. This killing event was to come to the attention of a key pioneer of 'mental maladies' as a medical specialism, **Jean-Etienne Esquirol** as well as the then King of France. Much later the event was also be used by eminent twentieth-century social thinker **Michel Foucault** as an example par excellence of how madness, and most if not all other phenomena including murder, cannot be understood without taking into account the comprehensive complexities of the social context in which it occurs and especially the enacting of power. From his position alternative comprehensions of madness to those of Esquirol, such as **Sigmund Freud**'s ingenious psychoanalytic inspection of the unconscious mind, either ignore or, in Freud's case, underplay the way in which society 'constructs' madness. In the twenty-first century, the case of Norwegian multiple murderer **Anders Breivik** also illustrates how madness continues to defy accurate description and broad agreement amongst and between the professionals and the public.

Chapter 2

At just about the same time as the Rivière event was occurring in France, **John Perceval**, son of assassinated British Prime Minister Spencer Perceval, was coming to the end of his three-year incarceration in English lunatic asylums. During his incarceration, Perceval wrote an elaborate description of his own mental condition, the conditions of the asylums in which he was placed, and the condition of his relationships with his 'controllers'. Perceval's narrative provides discernments about the practices of psychiatry at its birth, and he points to the workings of the unconscious mind long before Freud was born. The ideas of sociologists **Andrew Scull** and **Erving Goffman**, and biologist and anthropologist **Gregory Bateson**, point to how the asylum era involved control rather than care, how the asylums became 'total institutions', how these institutions allowed psychiatry to elevate substantially its standing as a medical specialty, and how early (and by implication later) 'scientific' insights into causation were/are wrong. Control over madness is highlighted further in the case of **Howard Dully** who in the USA during the middle of the twentieth century was institutionalised and lobotomised (by ice-pick) when he was 12 years of age.

Chapter 3

Mary Barnes was a nurse who became a painter, poet and writer. Diagnosed at the age of 30 with a psychotic disorder, her treatment, frequently forced, included insulin therapy, electro-convulsive-therapy (ECT), anti-psychotic medication and being placed in a padded cell. Subsequently, she became one of the first patients of **Ronald David Laing**, a renegade Scottish medical practitioner who was in the 1960s part of a disparate group known (misleadingly) as 'anti-psychiatry'. Laing and his collaborators regard medicalised madness (especially schizophrenia) as a reasonable reaction given the madness of their family dynamics. Barnes was encouraged to regress into childhood. This involved two years in bed, and indulging in a lot of faeces-smearing, some of which she used in her art. Another renegade psychiatrist **Thomas Szsaz** claims that 'mental illness is a myth' unless a specific mental disorder has an identifiable organic cause. Other challenges to the medical idea of madness come from clinical psychologist **Richard Bentall** who views medicalised madness not as an abnormality but part of the continuum of human performance. Another psychologist, David Rosenhan, claims that psychiatrists are not at all adept at recognising the boundaries between mental normality and abnormality. Welsh poet and writer **Gwyneth Lewis** uses her own experience to argue that depression is logical emotionally and should be embraced.

Chapter 4

Stephen Fry is a celebrated British polymath and entertainer. Fry's long-term struggles with madness (medicalised as manic-depression/bi-polar disorder) and many other aspects of his personal life have been discussed by him regularly and publically. However, celebrity, especially if sought and personal revelation, especially when abundant, may not be a personality trait, normal or abnormal, which is only or wholly derived from within the individual. Such characteristics for historian and social critic **Christopher Lasch** are indicative of a 'culture of narcissism'. Moreover, a narcissistic culture and the steep rise in the diagnosis of manic-depression may exemplify what social thinker and psychotherapist **Eric Fromm** suggests is the overall insanity of society. That notions of sanity and insanity sit not only in the individual but in the practices and beliefs of particular cultures has long been argued by such anthropologists as **Cecil Helman** and **Arthur Kleinman**. The cannibalistic conduct of Swift Runner, a nineteenth-century North American Cree supposedly possessed by the spirit of a monster, and subsequent diagnostic dissembling, indicate both the intermingling of culture and madness as well as the transmutability of psychiatry knowledge.

Chapter 5

American journalist **Susannah Cahalan** refers to her 'month of madness' in 2009 which, after much medical muddling, was recognised as being the result of a specific 'brain' disorder. 'W.L', a nineteenth-century English miner, succumbed to a terrible death from general paralysis of the insane, the terminal stage of syphilis. Since the discovery of the responsible bacterium and invention of antibiotic medication fatal insanity from syphilis is preventable. Such biological connections to madness serve to reinforce claims that neuroscience and genetics, along with evolutionary psychology/psychiatry, can and should underpin psychiatry as a science. Such claims are made by psychiatrist and geneticist **Peter McGuffin**. However, these claims can be accused of 'scientism' whereby only scientific knowledge can be considered legitimate knowledge. Neurologist **Steven Rose** and psychodynamic psychologist **Oliver James** argue that these claims are not even justifiable scientifically and that psychological and social factors cannot be dismissed. Neuroscientist **Raymond Tallis** doubts that the gaze of neuroscience is commensurate with the subjective experience of madness, and imputes evolutionary psychology/psychiatry as nonsense. A remedy for these antagonistic positions for sociologist **Nikolas Rose** is the synthesis of social scientific and scientific psychiatric ideas.

Summary

In this Introduction, the purpose and design of the book has been stated. These centre on the challenge of understanding madness through the analysis of a series of ideas which are applied to stories imparted by those who have been voted mad. Whether or not a realistic idea emerges from the application and analysis of these ideas is deliberated in the Conclusion.

No matter what judgement can be fashioned from the ideas, the stories are about real people who have endured or embraced (or both) their madness once so voted.

Notes

1 The idiom 'idea' as used in this book (along with 'theory', 'outlook', 'viewpoint', 'standpoint', etc.) encompasses personal and professional explanations of madness. An idea may be the result of or supported by individual insight (as with autobiographies), cogent argument, or empirical evidence (or a mixture or all of the types of 'evidence').
2 'Natural sciences' or simply 'science', in this context refers to the primary scientific subjects of biology, chemistry, engineering and physics. These sciences furnish the secondary sciences which are relevant to modern psychiatric medicine (and to a lesser degree psychology) especially genetics, neurology and biochemistry, along with related diagnostic technologies and treatments. I include psychology as a 'social science' alongside, for example, sociology and anthropology.
3 There are exceptions such as the occasional use of a court order to allow physicians to continue or curtail life-saving treatment against the wishes of their patient.

Further reading

Hirst, P., and Woolley, P. (1982) *Social Relations and Human Attributes*. London: Tavistock.

Porter, R. (1987) *A Social History of Madness: Stories of the Insane*. London: Weidenfeld & Nicolson.

Scull, A. (2015) *Madness in Civilisation: From the Bible to Freud, from the Madhouse to Modern Medicine*. London: Thames & Hudson.

1

MADNESS MANUFACTURED

Pierre Rivière

France, 3rd June 1835. A seemingly inconsequential 20-year-old peasant called Pierre Rivière was living in the seemingly inconsequential village of La Faucterie situated within the Normandy commune of Aunay. Yet, Rivière was to become a celebrated case study for one of France's most celebrated – and controversial – twentieth-century philosophers, Michel Foucault. Foucault's intellectual influence in the social sciences has endured, and much of his philosophical authority is built on his critiques of madness (Mills, 2003).

What had Rivière done to bring him to the attention of Foucault? The title of the intellectually pioneering book about Rivière published in 1975 by Foucault and his research team at the prestigious *Collège de France* is an indication as to why Rivière might have been considered unusual:

> I, Pierre Rivière, having slaughtered my mother, my sister, and my brother….

However, this multiple domestic murder, albeit one of such apparent ferocity (leaving vertebrae severed, skulls crushed, and brains slashed) and the victims being the killer's own pregnant mother and two of his siblings, was not at that time unusual. About 10 people per year in nineteenth-century France – which had half its current population – killed one or both parents and/or another close relative (parricide), or killed their spouse and one or more of their children and then possibly themselves (familicide). One study of the period 1991–2008 in France reports that there were only seven multiple slayings of a family by a member of the family, although in all of these cases it was the father, not a sibling who was the perpetrator (Makhlouf and Rambaud, 2014). Furthermore, during the violent history of humanity, there had been thousands of multiple murders and millions of single murders by 1975.

Even at the time, the case attracted the attention of those in the highest echelons of France's political and professional hierarchy. King Louis-Philippe I, who ruled France from 1830 to 1848, became involved, as did Jean-Etienne Dominique Esquirol, a physician who was France's senior specialist in mental medicine and one of the first in the world. Esquirol was in effect one of the world's first psychiatrists. He pioneered science in psychiatry and thereby the medicalisation of madness. He also promoted in France the large-scale segregation of the mad into institutions.

Moreover, a wider audience was introduced to this long-gone event with the release in 1976 of the art-house film *Moi, Pierre Rivière, ayant égorgé ma mère, ma soeur et mon frère...* (the title of Foucault's book in French) directed by René Allio. The film is naturalistic in the sense that the story is delivered at a routine everyday pace and most of the actors are villagers recruited from the area of Normandy in which the killings had taken place over 130 years previously. Since then Rivière's violent undertakings and Foucault's analysis of them continue to be aired. For example, Laurent Stéphan has performed in venues across France a one-man stage-play titled *Pierre Rivière, l'âme du crime* ('the soul of crime') depicting Foucault's consideration of the case. A second film about Rivière titled *Retour en Normandie* ('Back to Normandy'), this time directed by Nicolas Philibert who had been a young assistant director in the first film, was released in 2006. This second film revisits not only the happenings of 1835 but the making of René Allio's film. What Philibert does in his film is to interview and observe the 'actors' who had participated in Allio's film. This he does in their homes and at their place of work as well as in some of locations used in the original film. Superficially, it seems that Philibert is recording what the villagers in the main express as happy memories of their short-lived film careers. However, what is revealed subtly in *Retour en Normandie* is a deeper level of personal and social strife related to State power and how it affects the lives of those living in rural France during the twenty-first century, as well as issues concerning madness. All of which are implicitly compared with Rivière's situation in the nineteenth century.

To recap: attending to Rivière's deeds there are contemporaneously a host of local medical and legal practitioners, the monarch of a key country on the world-stage, and the most prominent physician of the mind in that country and in many others; subsequently a famed innovative thinker and his colleagues were to write a thought-provoking thesis on Rivière which was then to instigate the making of artistic portrayals of that thesis and the attention of countless social scientists.

What could be so intriguing? Surely this was a straightforward crime with an obvious killer? If anything at all needs further contemplation what could this be other than the veracity of these facts in the light of new factual evidence?

Crime scene

Taking the 'facts' as first presented by Foucault (1975), the scene of the crime was, as described by neighbours and the officials who were summoned, horrific but clear-cut. There were bodies, blood, and no indication that death had been caused other than through violence and which seemingly had not been conducted by any of the dead as can happen in some instances of familicide. The circumstantial evidence alone did not require elaborate detective work to determine culpability. Rivière's grandmother had come across the scene as it was unfolding and witnessed the slaying of her grand-daughter. The alarm is raised by the grandmother and Rivière drops the blood-stained weapon and removes himself from the scene just as neighbours and officials are starting to arrive. Rivière admits his guilt to two of his fellow villagers as he was leaving the vicinity.

Adding further weight to the obvious indications of his responsibility for this domestic carnage, many of those from the village in which he lived were to provide the authorities with incriminating declarations about his, in their view, odd and brutal predisposition. He had, they were to testify, a history when younger of idiocy and of cruelty to animals and children. Hence murderousness when older, these character witnesses affirmed, was hardly surprising.

After the killings, he stayed hidden in a nearby wood where he survived for a month on plants and roots. Rivière is seen acting oddly by locals living in the area of the wood and eventually law officers are summoned. He does not flee, however, on realising he has been recognised, and when arrested offers no resistance. Replying to the gendarmes when they queried where he was from (an odd first question as 'who are you?' would seem more appropriate) that he was 'from everywhere'. When then asked where he was going, he replies 'where God commands'.

Contrary confessions

Rivière is taken by his captors to their barracks in the town of Langannerie. According to the Report of the Sergeant of Gendarmerie at Langannerie, who asks why he has carried out the murders (a more pertinent question than 'where do you live?'), Rivière offers freely his motives. These are that his mother had sinned in the eyes of God because of her loathsome attitude towards her husband, and his brother and sister had sinned by taking her part in the parental dispute by deciding to stay living with their mother rather than, as he had done when the family split apart, gone to live with his father.

When interrogated on July 9th 1835, by the Examining Judge of the District of Vire, Exupere Legrain, he confesses once again and repeats that his actions had been dictated by God because of his father's familial predicament:

> Legrain: For what motive did you murder your mother, your sister Victoire and your brother Jules?

Rivière: Because God ordered me to justify His providence, they were
united.

Legrain: What do you mean by saying they were united?

Rivière: All three of them were in league to persecute my father.

Legrain and Rivière in Foucault, 1975, pp.19–20

The following day, again voluntarily, he provides the Examining Judge with
what he now states are the true reasons for his killings. In this second version
given to Legrain, he focuses again on the plight of his father as the reason for the
deaths but does not confer responsibility onto God but on himself. He says he
wishes to 'tell the truth' that he decided to kill the three members of his family
in order to alleviate his father from what he calls his (the father's) 'difficulties'.
Rivière continues:

> I wished to deliver him from an evil woman who had plagued him continually
> ever since she became his wife, who was ruining him, who was driving him
> to such despair that he was sometimes tempted to commit suicide.
>
> *Legrain and Rivière in Foucault, 1975, pp.23–24*

He repeats that he had killed his sister because she had sided with their
mother, but adds an extra detail when referring to why his brother had to die.
The brother had aligned himself with his mother against his father but he (the
brother) also 'loved' his mother and sister.

The Examining Judge reports that this second account by Rivière, which
encompasses details of his childhood, further information about his family
life, as well as elaboration on the killings, was delivered in an articulate and
methodical fashion which lasted two hours. Also, Rivière, when prompted by
the Examining Judge, expresses remorse that had he the opportunity he would
not repeat what he accepts readily as his 'crime'. Rivière states his feelings of
compunction surfaced not long after he had conducted his slayings.

> Yes, sir, an hour after my crime my conscience told me that I had done evil
> and I would not have done it over again.
>
> *Rivière in Foucault, 1975, p.38*

The question not seemingly considered by the Examining Judge when
interviewing Rivière is what triggered the remorse at that time? What had
changed in Rivière's mind and/or in his circumstances to lead him to express
regret? More importantly, what had changed for him to shift the locus of the
justification from implied madness to a declaration of badness? Remorse, if it
is gauged genuine, does usually preclude the particular psychiatric diagnoses of
psychopathy.[1]

The Examining Judge at the end of his interrogation of Rivière reads back
to him the transcription which has been recorded by an attendant scribe. The

Judge asks him if everything he (Rivière) has said and which then appears in the transcript is truthful, and if so would he put it all in his own handwriting. Rivière says it is and he will. He duly starts a few days later on what becomes an 11-day task expanding on what was contained in his second verbalised and transcribed confession. He produces an articulate and methodical document which is nearly 24,000 words long.

In the meantime the transcript from the interrogation of the Examining Judge provides substantial enough evidence for the District Prosecutor Royal at the Civil Court of Vire to support a submission to the Royal Court at Caen, sitting as a pre-trial hearing. The evidence is a summary by the District Prosecutor of statements supplied by Rivière's father, grandmother and that of another sister of Rivière.

In the summary, there is mention of Rivière having been from birth a problem to his family due to his taciturn and obstinate manner, the absence of noticeable affection towards both his parents but particularly his hostility towards his mother. Also referred to is his pleasure in killing animals and threatening to do the same to his peers, his night-time dealings with the devil, and his dislike of all women. Less incriminatingly, mention is made of him being literate (illiteracy was not uncommon amongst the peasantry in nineteenth-century France: Charle, 1994), and that he particularly enjoyed reading about philosophy and religion.

Notwithstanding literacy, the District Prosecutor is convinced of Rivière's guilt. He sides, however, with 'badness' rather than 'madness' to explain his motives for murder. In particular, he discounts a diagnosis of monomania, a now-defunct psychiatric category invented by Esquirol to account for why otherwise normal nineteenth-century French people may have a moment of madness:

> [Rivière] … is not a religious monomaniac as he tried to make out at first; nor is he an idiot, as some witnesses seemed to suppose him to be … [H]e stifled the voice of conscience and did not struggle hard enough to control the propensities of his evil character.
>
> *District Prosecutor Royal in Foucault, 1975, p.40*

There is, however, a contradiction in the District Prosecutor's opinion. Stating that Rivière followed the promptings of evil for his cruelty implies an uncontrollable impulse rather than a conscious and voluntary choice. The District Prosecutor seems to want to have Rivière punished (the death penalty) for not being psychologically strong enough to control his susceptibility to being bad.

Uncontrollable (or irresistible) impulses are an element of Esquirol's monomania. Another subdivision of monomania apart from the 'religious monomania' mentioned by the District Prosecutor, is homicidal monomania. The homicidal monomaniac, asserts Esquirol, has an intact reason and conscience and an irresistible urge to kill:

These maniacs perceive, compare and judge correctly; but they are drawn aside, from the slightest cause and even without object, to the commission of acts of violence and fury.

Esquirol, 1845, p.362

The ability of 'these maniacs' to think logically about their actions and comprehend the moral worth of those actions is, argues Esquirol, at times, overridden by their emotions with disastrous consequences for them and their targets.

At the meeting of the pre-trial on 25 July 1835 at the Royal Court at Caen, at which the District Prosecutor reports and Rivière's memoir is submitted, it is decided that the weight of the evidence is sufficient for the accusation of homicide to be recommended to the Regional Prosecutor at Caen. This is on the basis that Rivière did with malice aforethought kill his mother, brother and sister. The Court comments that the evidence indicates he has neither memory loss nor is his intellect is damaged. The recommendation is accepted by the Regional Prosecutor.

The memoir

Beginning on 10 July and ending on 21 July, Rivière had written his long and lucid memoir whilst in gaol awaiting trial. He details his childhood and provides his version of the incidents which had been described by witnesses from the village as evidence of his cruelty, and provides particulars of the frequently tense and occasionally malicious relationship between his mother and father. According to Rivière's memoir, his parents, who married in 1813 so that his father could avoid military service, had never been compatible. Their incompatibility led his mother, along with various relatives and Rivière's sister and brother, to live in one house, and his father with Pierre in another three miles away. This arrangement did not prevent his father having, according to Rivière, his passive disposition imposed on by the mother's oppressive personality. Disagreements were common and often focused on petty disagreements over finances, furniture and food. These disagreements for Rivière were largely provoked by his mother to provide opportunities for her to torment his father rather than being about the subject over which they ostensibly were arguing.

Rivier's negative opinion about women generally is exhibited in his memoir and seems to have derived from his personal construal of Christian scripture, which in adolescence he had taken to reading avidly. He expresses the horror of incest and bestiality and his dread of contact with human and animal females. Sex with blood-relatives and beasts was his greatest worry but sex with anyone or anything was also perturbing:

[C]arnal passion troubled me: I believed that it was unworthy of me ever to think of indulging in it. Above all I had a horror of incest, which caused me to shun approaching the women in my family.

Rivière in Foucault, 1975, p.102

For Rivière women had, following the French Revolution in 1789, managed to take from men their dominance in society. What he wanted was a return to the ancient Roman social hierarchy in which fathers had the right to decide on the life and death of their wives and children.

In his memoire Rivière reaffirms that it was he who took the lives of his mother, sister and brother:

> My brother Jule had come back from school. Taking advantage of this opportunity I seized the bill [a pruning implement], I went into my mother's house and I committed that fearful crime, beginning with my mother, then my sister and my little brother, after that I struck them again and again.
>
> *Rivière in Foucault, 1975, p.112*

Rivière also reaffirms his guilt and refers to his remorse which he says he first experienced when reaching the forest at Aunay where he went after the killings:

> I regained my full senses … ah can it be so, I asked myself, monster that I am! Hapless victims! Can I possibly have done that, no it is but a dream! Ah but it is all too true! … I wept … I fell to the ground.
>
> *Rivière in Foucault, 1975, p.113*

Hence, there was no dispute over Rivière's culpability before, during, or after the trial by any of those associated with the case, including Rivière. But there was, and still is, debate over his mental state.

Mad–bad–normal

Rivière's various statements about his motives contribute to the debate about his psychological disposition. At different points, he indicates madness, badness and normality. Initially, he claimed to have seen visions and heard voices (from God) which led him to believe God wanted him to kill. These and similar conceptions and perceptions contemporary psychiatrists consider misconceptions (delusions) and misperceptions (hallucinations) are 'positive' signs of severe mental disorder, probably schizophrenia (Royal College of Psychiatrists, 2015). This necessitates adjudication by psychiatrists on God's intentions. That is, psychiatrists are assuming God, should he/she exist, would not have wanted such unpleasant outcomes as happened to this peasant family and therefore such discernments and sensations are false. However, if God does not exist then the issue of who is mad has much wider implications.

In the second version of his confession, Rivière formulates a scenario of enduring unjust and damaging family dynamics, which he suggests had been especially detrimental to his father. It was this unfairness, Rivière declares, that drove him to eradicate the person he held responsible for its instigation (his mother). His sister had to die because she had collaborated with her mother in making their father's life a misery. In explaining why his brother had to die he offers yet another reason to those already provided in earlier confessions. Besides the brother siding with and loving the mother his fate was sealed because he was very much loved by his father. Therefore, if Rivière only killed the father's prime tormentors he feared that his father may well forgive him. By also killing the brother Rivière believed the father would so abhor his murderous actions then he would rejoice in him being convicted and also would not feel guilty about having somehow allowed such a terrible event to take place within his family. Hence, it can be argued that rather than madness triggering such extreme action to deal with this seemingly woeful state of family affairs, it could only come about if the person was evil. 'Badness' could only be the prime cause of this calculated decision. However, it could also be argued that what Rivière states regarding his childhood, his family and why he killed, implies that any otherwise normal person could have behaved in a similar 'evil' fashion if placed in similar circumstances.

Therefore, Rivière's accounts of his killings imply two contrary interpretations: (a) his actions were the consequence of not being fully in charge of his mental faculties and thereby was not responsible for them; (b) his actions were premeditated and malevolent and hence he was responsible for them. However, this dichotomy is simplistic. Questions relating to the mental state of any murderer of interest to defence and prosecution lawyers, expert psychiatric witnesses and theorists of criminality, may include: is the killer mad or bad?; whether mad or bad, what made him/her so?; is it because the killer is a 'faulty' individual', because he/she is or was living in a 'faulty society', or is it a mixture of the two 'faults'?; if the killer is mad, what type of madness does he/she have?; for example, is the killer psychotic or a psychopath?; if the latter, why is it that many theorists of crime and some psychologists and psychiatrists, do not believe it is an authentic mental disorder but a category in which the courts, either following or rejecting 'expert' advice, may place those who do not fit easily into either the categories of badness or madness (Bonn, 2014); could it be that he/she was/is a bit of both?; no matter what madness the killer has, was it relevant to the killing; might it be that the killer was, and is, sane but put in an insane situation and any normal person might have killed if placed in similar circumstances?

Not only murder but many, perhaps all, aspects of human performance, may well have a similarly complicated matrix of predisposing and precipitating causative factors. Furthermore, complexity abounds in the shaping of how causation is conceived. Personal, professional, political, economic and military contexts, to a greater or lesser degree influence which cause is considered if indeed causation is considered at all.

The medical practitioner who first examined Rivière did so soon after his arrest on 21 July 1835, and his view was adopted by the prosecution. This was a generalist physician, Dr Bouchard. Bouchard was definite in his conclusion that Rivière was not mad. However, his justification for diagnosing Rivière not mad is peppered with connotations of his (Rivière's) impending or perceptible madness. For example, Bouchard ascribes Rivière's killings to a momentary period of 'over-excitement', and regards him as having 'dark' and 'obsessive' ideas regarding his father's predicament. Bouchard also mentions how Rivière shunned his community, and that he seemed extraordinarily calm when describing the killings. Moreover, Bouchard suggests that Rivière has a particular type of disposition which harks back to ancient medical ideas about personality types based on 'humors':

> He shows every sign of a bilious-melancholic temperament.
>
> *Bouchard in Foucault, 1975, p.122*

So what meaning or meanings can be attached to the notion of a 'bilious-melancholic' temperament? In Greco-Roman medicine it means a mixture of persistent introversion, worrying, particular preoccupations, and periodic bouts of aggression (Peterson, 1982). But from a non-medical viewpoint it could be taken as implying that Rivière was mostly miserable and occasionally bad-tempered. If adopting contemporary diagnostic categories from psychiatry (bearing in mind that these do change with each revamped version of the two main classification systems) he might be diagnosed with for example, clinical depression, anxiety, compulsive-obsessive-disorder, manic-depression (bipolar disorder), and/or intermittent explosive disorder.

There would at first to be no such vacillation in Dr Vastel's opinion. Vastel, a physician attached to one of the largest mental asylums in France (the Bon Sauveur in Paris) claimed to have studied the mental state of 11,000 madmen which by any standards would infer a high degree of proficiency in being able to separate accurately who was mad, who was bad and who was neither. He examined Rivière on 25 October 1835 after receiving a request from Rivière's father and the lawyer for the defence. The father and defence lawyer were asserting that Rivière had been mad all along. They especially wanted to emphasise that he was so at the time of the killings. What the father hoped for was a medical diagnosis to support a plea of insanity to ensure that his son, should he be found culpable, was not executed. Rivière's declared tactic of killing his brother to ensure his father was implacably unsympathetic towards him had patently not worked. After reviewing the documents relating to the case including the memoir written by Rivière and his own observations of the prisoner, Vastel is completely convinced that he is insane:

> [T]he act which the prosecution considered to be an atrocious crime was simply the deplorable result of true mental alienation … Truly, I have never seen a more manifest case of insanity among the hundreds of monomaniacs I have treated.
>
> *Vastel in Foucault, 1975, pp.127–131*

The term 'mental alienation' was a commonly used synonym for madness/ mental disorder and medical practitioners who specialised in matters of the mind were known as 'alienists' (Porter, 2003). However, Vastel is borrowing Esquirol's particular diagnostic category of monomania. Monomania is characterised by a partial state of madness in which one or more aspects of the will, intellect and emotions are afflicted, but the rest of the individual's performance is normal. For Esquirol and Vastel monomania was usually a disorder of heredity but which required a trigger such as sudden death of a loved one, financial ruin or interpersonal strife.

Rivière had, according to Vastel, religious delusions along with delusions regarding his family. Vastel also accommodates in his diagnosis Rivière's shifts in his confessions. These changes, argues Vastel, exemplify psychological derangement, not cogent calculation – that is, madness not badness. Vastel admits that Rivière may appear to be sane but argues that even if this was so then it is likely only to be temporary, and he remains dangerous to himself and society and should be kept imprisoned. This is not a consistent position as how can Vastel argue both that Rivière is definitely mad and then accept that he may not be? His contention that Rivière was mad at the time of the killing and probably still is but certainly will be again is not helped by the defendant's persistent claims that he is not mad but bad and deserves to be executed.

Vastel's opinion, which challenged that of Bouchard, was in turn challenged by Bouchard. Bouchard contended that Rivière was not a monomaniac and that any delusion he might have was not focused on one issue. Bouchard also disputed other possible diagnoses of madness. Despite Bouchard earlier stating that Rivière's over-excitement had been a factor in causing him to kill, he argues that a diagnosis of mania (characterised by excitement albeit to excess) was self-evidently wrong as Rivière was not regularly agitated. Despite many if not most of those who knew Rivière well arguing the reverse, Bouchard claims that it was also self-evident that he wasn't an idiot as he could read and write and there was no clinical evidence of brain damage.

Bouchard was, however, somewhat out-of-date (so too was Vastel) as far as his understanding of monomania was concerned. The inventor of the idea of monomania, Esquirol, had by then altered his description of it. He had removed the requirement for a diagnosis of monomania which necessarily includes intellectual disturbance. That is, Esquirol's new position on monomania was that where there are disturbances of the emotions the intellect may not necessarily be affected. The homicidal monomaniac may be driven by some unknowable force of heredity but his/her reason remains sound and therefore no delusions at all may be found.

Faced with the disparity of opinions between Bouchard and Vastel, the trial judge called for further expert medical opinion from a Dr Trouvé and a Dr Lebidois. It is hard to identify exactly what opinion these later two doctors provided, and there may have been views sought from further aspiring experts. In total, 13 witnesses were called by the prosecution and nine for the defence.

The judge and the jury were faced with an equal split between those who argued Rivière was sane and those who argued he was insane.

The verdict

The jury, which included two medical practitioners and two lawyers, various property owners and a wine merchant, deliberated for three hours. They returned a unanimous verdict of guilty to parricide. Their verdict implied that they believed Rivière to be bad and not mad. The punishment was to be execution.

However, the steadfastness of the jury's decision, as with medical opinion, had imperfections. Half of the jury, comprising 12 men, expressed openly their belief that the evidence that had been given at the trial indicated Rivière had never been fully sane and that there were extenuating circumstances. Moreover, a petition was organised by a majority of the jury in support of the death penalty being commuted to life imprisonment. The petition was reinforced by the trial judge's recommendation in his report for the exercise of royal prerogative for such a change to the punishment.

A formal appeal was lodged in November 1835 with the Criminal Division of the Court of Cassation, France's court of last resort which adjudicates on interpretations of the law. Rivière had to sign the appeal to be accepted at the Court of Cassation. He did sign but reluctantly because he agreed with both the verdict and the punishment. Although the appeal failed, the petition continued to collect supportive evidence, including yet more medical opinions. Especially useful to the petitioners were the opinions of Dr Marc, the 'Court Physician to His Majesty' and that of Esquirol who both stated that Rivière was insane. Moreover, they observed that given Rivière's previous behaviour he should have been placed in confinement much earlier in his life as he had been 'too ill' to remain at large.

Succumbing to the pressure brought by the petitioners and medical luminaries, the Minister of Justice in February 1836 submitted a report to the King in which he refers to the disputes over material evidence and the 'doctors' conflicting reports'. The Minister proposes that the King's royal prerogative should be applied to commute the punishment of death to life-long 'penal servitude'. The King agreed. Rivière was sent to the Central Prison at Beaulieu in March 1836 for life.

Rivière's life sentence lasted only until 20 October 1840. On that day he committed suicide by hanging.

The prison report on Rivière's suicide refers to 'unmistakable signs of madness' (quoted in Foucault, 1975, p.171). The report also comments that Rivière had for some time regarded himself as already dead, and had to be placed in solitary confinement because he had threatened to kill fellow prisoners and warders if they did not cut off his head.

Jean-Etienne Esquirol

Jean-Etienne Dominique Esquirol (1772–1840) was intent on investigating insanity meticulously, and his work was to have a considerable impact on how madness became understood and dealt with in the nineteenth century throughout Europe. Moreover, he helped to plant the (scientific) seeds for what has become the dominant perspective for over two centuries throughout the West and increasingly globally – that psychiatry has obtained or will find the real answers to the realities of madness.

For Esquirol, madness is a disorder of the brain which altered the normal functioning of thinking, feeling and behaving. In his collected works titled *Mental Maladies: Treatise on Insanity*, published posthumously in 1845, he defines insanity thus:

> Insanity or mental alienation is a cerebral affection, ordinarily chronic and without fever; characterised by disorders of sensibility, understanding, intelligence and will.
>
> *Esquirol, 1845, p.21*

Esquirol's conceptualisation of madness became the principle underlying medical interest in the scientific study of madness in French universities.

Cerebral Centricity

However, Germany was to lead the way in the scientific study specifically of the brain as the primary locus of madness through the efforts of physician Wilhelm Griesinger (1817–1868). Griesinger was in 1845 to become Professor of Psychiatry and Neurology at Berlin University (Haas, 1997).

Esquirol campaigned for the medical profession to be the legitimate managers of madness within the confines the asylum and for the asylums to serve as a form of treatment. Along with being confined, crude, some of which currently may be considered as cruel, physical methods of treatments were proffered if not imposed (Porter, 1987). These included enemas, emetics, bloodletting, spinning chairs and cold baths. Similarly, Griesinger believed in medicalising madness and medical dominance. He justified his position by claiming that the brain was central to understanding madness and his profession was central to understanding the brain:

> Insanity being a disease, and that disease being an affection of the brain, it can therefore only be studied in a proper manner from the medical point of view.
>
> *Griesinger, 1882; original 1867, p.7*

Griesinger also encouraged incarceration, but he was in favour of early discharge when the patient's mental state and social circumstances allowed. He has become recognised as one of the founders of community care as a policy (Rössler and Meise, 1994).

Esquirol's motives in recommending incarceration were laudable (as were Griesinger's). He had observed poverty-stricken mad people living in lamentable conditions. He also wanted medical practitioners to be involved in caring for the criminally insane. That is, on philanthropic as well as professional ethical grounds, he even regarded those people who had committed murder, and who could be classified as not responsible by reason of insanity, deserving of medical treatment rather than legal punishment. The latter could be a death sentence. There is, therefore, no fundamental contradiction or immovable impediment preventing the most biological-minded and professionally dominating psychiatrist from being a social reformer and a decent human.

In 1817 Esquirol initiated what was probably the first formal teaching about 'maladies mental' in the dining-room of his place of work, the Salpêtrière hospital in Paris. Esquirol, using his own money, at his own expense, toured around France, examining facilities for the mad. He learned that these facilities, where available, were inadequate to say the least:

> I have seen them naked, clad in rags, having but straw to shield them from the cold humidity of the pavement where they lie. I have seen them coarsely fed, leacking [sic] air to briethe [sic], water to quench their thirst, wanting the basic necessities of life.
>
> *Esquirol quoted in Weiner, 1994, p.234*

If not in these dire conditions then the mad could be found at mercy of brutal supervision chained in filthy and lightless dungeons or caverns where they would be treated worse than wild beasts.

Esquirol lobbied the relevant senior politician (the Minister of Interior), and wrote a series of articles, arguing for reform throughout France. The reform he wanted and achieved was to spread what was already happening in Paris, the building of specialist hospitals for the mad (asylums) and the development of mad-doctoring within those institutions. Asylums were to become the main means to manage the mad, and madness was to be medicalised.

Most of the medical treatments prescribed by Esquirol and the other asylum-based medical practitioners were makeshift and some were fearsome. But, Esquirol didn't just blithely administer the leech and purgative. He attempted to assess their worth in treating particular conditions and did so methodically given that methods of assessment were also rudimentary. Furthermore, although Esquirol (1845) wanted and got medical dominance over the mad, he also advocated a 'law of love' and a 'moral regime'. Griesinger (1882) recommended 'cupping', ice to the head and opium, but he also admired the pioneers of the openly more humane 'moral therapy' approach, the French physician Philippe Pinel (Weiner, 1992) and the English businessman and Quaker William Tuke (Kabria and Metcalfe, 2014).

Equirol's understanding of causation is relatively refined, that is relative to the state of scientific ideas about madness at the time. In many aspects, they also stand the test of time. The interplay between heredity, biology, emotional and physical trauma and the social-environment are all in his *Mental Maladies* (as they are in Griesinger's writings). He recognises that the causes of 'mental alienation' are numerous and varied and only a deeper insight into genetic and social factors is absent:

> [Causes] … are general or specific, physical or moral, primitive or secondary, predisposing or exciting. Not only do climates, seasons, age, sex [he refers later to both gender and sexuality, with erotomania and masturbation scrutinised in particular], temperament, profession and mode of life [he clarifies this later as lifestyle and social class], have an influence upon the frequency, character, duration, crises, and treatment of insanity; but this malady is still modified by laws, civilisation, morals, and the political condition of people.
>
> *Esquirol, 1845, p.30*

There are, in Esquirol's *Mental Maladies,* chapters on symptoms and types of madness: hallucinations; illusions; fury; epilepsy (regarded then as a form of insanity either in its own right or alongside other forms); melancholy (that is, depression); demonomania (the delusion of being possessed by evil spirits or the devil); suicide; mania; dementia; idiocy (included as type of insanity); and monomania.

Griesinger had his own version of monomania, arguing that madness was chiefly the consequence of a single brain disorder, a unitary psychosis (*einheitspsychose*), but Esquirol's unitary category was much more well-known during the nineteenth century.

Monomania was Esquirol's great discovery, or so he thought. As with many historical ideas about madness, badness and normality, there are parallels with the twenty-first century. Monomania resonates with what later became known as psychopathic disorder (and later still 'anti-social personality disorder') whereby some of those classified as such perform perhaps at a high level of intelligence and functionality at work and in their family lives, but also carry out one or many heinous acts. What also resonates today is Esquirol's conviction that there was a hereditary cause, albeit for him 'unknowable'.

Warrior gene

Esquirol can therefore can be applauded for incredible foresight because by the 21st century the idea of genes determining behaviour is giving credence to what has become known as 'neurolaw' (Goodenough and Zeki, 2006). Neurolaw refers to a controversial line of defence in criminal cases. For example, it has been argued that the so-called 'Warrior Gene' which leads to a deficiency in a particular brain chemical (the neurotransmitter-metabolising enzyme monoamine oxidase A – MAOA), can be linked to aggressive outbursts as it was in this Italian case:

> An Italian court has cut the sentence given to a convicted murderer by a year because he has genes linked to violent behaviour — the first time that behavioural genetics has affected a sentence passed by a European court.
>
> *Feresin, 2009*

The courts' decision referred to the work of Pietro Pietrini, a molecular neuroscientist at Italy's University of Pisa, and Giuseppe Sartori, a cognitive neuroscientist at the University of Padova. They had carried out a series of brain-imaging scans and genetic tests on the killer and believed they had identified abnormalities which have in the relevant research literature been associated with violent behaviour. These abnormalities included the 'Warrior Gene'. However, the notion that some people have a specific inherited combatant component is highly controversial (Powledge, 2014).

James Fallon is a renowned neuroscientist known for his work on particular structural and genetic abnormalities in the brains of psychopaths, many of whom are killers. After many years researching the subject he was to discover that he has most of these abnormalities including the 'Warrior Gene' (Hagerty, 2010). So far he has not been diagnosed as a psychopath nor admitted to killing anyone. This would seem to dilute the proposition of a direct and overriding link which could qualify as a strong defence in murder trials.

However, even if a gene or genes for psychopathic murdering was discovered then much more evidence would have to be ascertained to explain its or their precise significance in the convoluted interplay of other biological factors, conscious control and especially social contexts. For example, Central America has a much higher rate of homicide than Europe. Does that mean that there is a genetic difference between the two groups of people which leads to this disparity in the homicide figures? A much more obvious variation is the respective traditions, cultures and in particular living conditions.

What Fallon argues is that his genetic theory is not redundant but remains robust. There are other factors in his background, he suggests, such as the normative effect of his loving family and the diversionary benefit of his academic career which have, so far, prevented him from becoming a psychopathic killer (Fallon, 2014). What Fallon, so far, has not done is to kill his theory. Many of the types of and explanations for madness, including monomania, formed by the founders of psychiatry are no longer coveted by psychiatrists today. Many of today's types and explanations may not be coveted in the future.

However, despite the variability over what is accepted as a legitimate idea, is the general direction taken to try to understand madness one of progress and is this progress in the hands of psychiatry? Alternatively, does each historical epoch and/or societal set-up produce its own meaning of madness and may this meaning be provided by disciplines other than that of psychiatry? Michel Foucault and his colleagues address this dilemma.

Michel Foucault

Paul Michel Foucault (1926–1984) was not medically trained but he did have a lot to say about doctors. He had become in the 1970s Professor of the History of Systems of Thought at the prestigious *Collège de France* specialising in, amongst many other topics, medical thinking. He and his colleagues who edited and contributed to *I, Pierre Rivière, having slaughtered my mother, my sister, and my brother*…. supply their thoughts on the way in which Rivière's mental state had been interpreted by purported medical experts as well as by Rivière. They also offer their own interpretations about the case. What is supplied in that book, therefore, is a collection of competing discourses identified by Foucault and his colleagues.

Discourse and power

For Foucault, Rivière's episode was not merely a sorrowful saga of one man's muddled mind no matter how complex the reasons for the muddle which led to murder. Foucault grasped that the case was unique because as well as the new judicial doctrine of extenuating circumstances being introduced at this point, this was the first opportunity to allow medical testimony to be formally introduced into the French courts specifically for the assessment of the condition of the accused's mind. Therefore, this was an important historical occasion in criminal justice and psychiatric practice. It was the onset of the continued and often rocky marriage of medical and legal opinion concerning criminality and madness. It, argued Foucault, marked a momentous shift in the way in which madness was regarded and regulated.

Medical authority over madness was expanding decidedly and mainly doing so within the confines of the asylum. Whilst this newly found power over a large proportion of human performance was sanctioned and fostered by the State, for Foucault it had been initiated and was being 'enjoyed' by medical practitioners. The introduction of their self-acclaimed knowledge about the pathologies of the mind into courts of law signified and reinforced medical authority over madness. What these additional (to the lawyers) experts to the criminal justice system required was a different way of referring to mad offenders which marked-out 'criminal insanity' as their territory. That is, they needed additional clinical concepts and clinical procedures, and a novel linguistic style, for what was to become a power-laden psychiatric 'discourse'.

The documents Foucault examined about the case disclosed contradictory opinions over various 'facts' surrounding the killings especially those concerning Rivière's intellectual capacity, the significance of his childhood deeds of contended cruelty, and his scale of culpability. Moreover, there were inconsistencies between those who considered Rivière mad regarding what madness he had.

Foucault argues that the differing viewpoints about Rivière's mental state indicate that Rivière's madness was not only understood inadequately but also demonstrates doubt about the whole notion of madness. The line of questioning which Foucault explored and answered so innovatively included: what is madness? is it a real or fabricated concept and condition; if not real then how and by whom has it been manufactured?

The happenings before, during and after the killings, have diverse interpretations and re-interpretations. Contending explanations are generated by him about his motivation because inevitably what he experiences in his mind does not (indeed cannot for him or anyone else) replicate exactly what others regard as reality. Hence, both what he did think and what he thinks when he reflects on what he thought will be different. Subsequently, what he verbalises about what he thought either to himself or to those to whom he confesses will produce further variations. On top of these variations, his thoughts produce mutations when they are written down for him and when he writes them down. Moreover, when the person supplying an account of an event is also the main participant then there are likely to be further disparities when compared to accounts supplied by observers. Whether an account is by a participant or observer (and all observers to some extent are participants), verbal or written, summarised or maximised, it will be idiosyncratic. Reality, therefore, appears to disappear in this multi-layered morass of impressions. That there is a reality containing real events which can be known and described accurately and perpetually is challenged by Foucault. Intriguingly, it has also come to be doubted by quantum physicists (Vedral, 2010).

These interpretative complexities and suspect affiliation to a knowable reality apply to all of those who gave an opinion on the Rivière case. This is so, according to Foucault, no matter how authoritatively the narrative in question is avowed as the truth. Foucault's point is that diagnostic uncertainty is not a matter of inadequate medical expertise but about certainty regarding mental (or physical) disorder not being possible – then or today.

Any particular discourse Foucault figures in the Rivière book, and in earlier publications (Foucault, 1961; 1963; 1966), is the outcome of the power wielded by the group it represents, and once established the discourse then further legitimises and reinforces that power. The discourse and resultant power of politicians, spiritual leaders, bankers, corporate directors and lawyers, will have been gained through actions likely to have a long and complex history to them, as it has been with the medical profession. Although a discourse operates at the level of interpersonal interactions, it is connected to wider social process. For example, the building of the asylums in the nineteenth century connects with the rise of psychiatry.

Domination by a particular group can be challenged or supported by other groups. In the domain of health and illness (physical and mental), clinical psychology may compete or comply with psychiatry, and a burgeoning array of therapies (for example, hypnosis, homoeopathy, acupuncture and naturopathy) either complement or provide an alternative to the services of the medical practitioner. What each group is attempting is the construction of a 'truth' which it alone is responsible for revealing and maintaining. Physicists, physicians and Popes proclaim that they have distinct understandings, some of which are construed as infallible. These alleged superior insights are meant to be the root of the power of the scientist, shaman, and Ayatollah, and his/her right to preach about the workings of the natural and supernatural worlds, and the performance of the living and the dead.

Foucault and his colleagues give their own interpretations in *I, Pierre Rivière, having slaughtered my mother, my sister, and my brother*.... What is supplied in that book, therefore, is a collection of competing discourses identified by Foucault and his colleagues and superimposed upon these are further discourses manufactured by them. Some of these superimposed interpretations steer into such outlandish claims on what was 'real' that in contrast they make those Foucault and his colleagues are critiquing appear much more reasonable as far as having any grasp on reality is concerned.

It is a premise of Foucault's understanding of history in much of his work that it cannot be understood retrospectively and that finding the 'facts' about people and events at any point historically can never be any more than finding a particular story which serves a particular purpose. This is an innovative but incongruous position for Foucault to take as he presents this position and many others as though they are facts. He searches for and professes to find, frequently without due diligence, facts (that is empirical evidence) to support his claims.

Ancien Régime

Jean-Pierre Peter and Jeanne Favret (in Foucault, 1975), members of Foucault's research team at the *Collège de France*, argue that Rivière's killings need to be understood not only or even at all as the crimes of an individual. For them, his killings had to be comprehended in the context of much social conflict. In particular, it was indicative of the subjugation of the peasantry. To back these two propositions there does seem to be some historical deposition.

What was France like in the early part of the nineteenth century according to orthodox historians? Christophe Charle (1994), Professor of History at the University of Paris (1994) in his exhaustive coverage of the social history of nineteenth-century France pays due respect to the complex business of making sense of the people and events and thereby avoids undue generalisations and assumptions. However, he does appear to believe in facts. What he shows is that the lot of the peasants in the decades after the 1789 French Revolution was not substantially different to how it had been for previous centuries within the feudal *ancien régime*. During the time of Pierre Rivière, benefits in what was ostensibly a more equitable social system were materialising in terms of food production and distribution, the control of plague and improved general health. However, the condition of peasant life varied considerably in different regions of France, within regions and between the cities and the provinces.

The first half of the nineteenth century was, according to Charle 'The Age of the Nobles'. The hierarchy remained rigid and oppressive, and dominated by the nobility with the King at the top and the peasantry remaining at the bottom. The latter were, suggests Charle, in effect still no more than serfs. Although divine right had been abolished, the King was still involved directly with most of the key political decision-making. There were periodic food crises and lethal epidemics. The latter was not helped by the deficient condition of both urban and rural housing, the absence of effective drainage and waste disposal, limited medical services in the countryside, and unwholesome personal hygiene. Bodily cleansing of any sort was not a priority for much of the populace.

Not only had the basis of political power not altered profoundly, but wealth inequality had not changed much since before the Revolution. Traders, bankers and administrators of the political regime, were joining the ranks of the very wealthy. However, rather than a money-economy taking over, wealth and power continued to be tied to land ownership.

The King of France, Louis-Philippe and his ministers declared a commitment to religious and political tolerance and social reform. There was a new constitution in 1830 whereby all Frenchmen (but not Frenchwomen) were to be equal before the law regardless of their rank. The number of those allowed to vote increased, but this still covered only a tiny minority of the population. Frenchwomen did not get suffrage until 1944.

France suffered from the consequences of rapid and uncontrolled urbanisation because of emerging industrialisation. There was a rise in crime, overcrowding, disease and examples of extreme destitution and social exclusion when work could not be found. Furthermore, the social fabric of French society had been damaged severely by the loss of 1.5 million people from 1789–1815 as a consequence of the Revolution, and the subsequent civil wars and the period of 'The Terror' during which tens of thousands of people were executed. What also is found at this time is the centrality of violence which was perpetually underneath the surface or spilt over into actual bloodshed due to the social conflicts between the established elite and groups vying to join its rank, and between the peasantry and urban workers.

There are, therefore, historical connections of French revolutionary violence and State power to the Rivière's murders. Punishments for acts that threatened the social order also alter. For example, the guillotine is replaced by the noose. The exploitative French nobility set the stage for violent (and murderous and self-destructive) responses by the peasantry.

For Peter and Favret, Rivière's killings represented a boil which had come to the surface and burst on a body riddled with an angry and pervasive sepsis. The boil, therefore, is only a symptom of an underlying disorder. Rivière's carnage denotes an inevitable outpouring of social pus. Hence, to focus only on the pathology of the boil will lead to nothing more than a superficial if not completely false analysis. Peter and Favret contend that Rivière is not a monster or madman, but a 'native terrorist'. That is, his actions are a forerunner of an uprising by the peasantry against those with power in France.

Neil Websdale (2013), Professor of Criminology at Northern Arizona University, in his exploration of the causes of familicide, offers an explanation extrapolated from the work of sociologist Norbert Elias. For Websdale, Rivière's murderousness was an example of the undoing of social constraints on basic human emotions after hundreds of years of conditioning thought the civilising process associated with Western civilisation.

Moreover, Peter and Favret, argue that Rivière's wish to have his death penalty carried out should have been allowed. For them Rivière's wanting to die should not have been countered by what they consider was his oppressor's hypocritical humanism and paternalism, aided and abetted by those medical practitioners setting their professional sights on establishing themselves as the prevailing authority on the workings of the mind. That is, his rights, including the right to perform self-murder, were being transcended by those of the State and the medical profession. The transcendence of an individual's autonomy over his/her life, with or without assistance, continues to the present time in many countries (Lewis, 2015).

For Blandine Barret-Kreigel, another of Foucault's collaborators on *I, Pierre Rivière, having slaughtered my mother, my sister, and my brother….*, murder is not only a serious act of illegality but any murder of a parent is more serious as it challenges the social order. France's social hierarchy in the nineteenth century was based on 'the family'. Ultimately in this social order, the King is considered the head of all families. Therefore, regicide is the crime-of-crimes, with the killing of any parent an implicit threat to this arrangement. The representatives of the criminal justice system throughout France, the King's personal legal and political entourage, and the King himself, all had an agenda of controlling parricide because of its link to regicide and the social order.

Foucault's argument that conditions, incidents, and people associated with madness (or murder) cannot be understood outside of their social context and in particular how power is organised in that context does seem to resonate with what happened on 3 June 1835 at the village of La Fauctcrie. That this can lead to questioning of the reality of madness and even murder, and by implication all reality, is itself questionable.

Madness and civilisation

However, Foucault had committed himself to the deconstruction of reality, which was to become the bedrock principle of social constructionist (Berger and Luckman, 1966) and postmodernist perspectives (Derrida, 1967) long before he analysed Pierre Rivière. His most famous book on madness titled *Madness and Civilisation* was published originally in 1961 (with the title *Histoire de la folie à l'âge classique*) which is long before the publication of *I, Pierre Rivière*. In *Madness and Civilisation* there is the theoretical framework through which he would later analyse Rivière and his circumstances. This is despite Foucault insisting in *I, Pierre Rivière* that there would be no interpretation of the case by him and his colleagues.

Foucault in *Madness and Civilisation* already is arguing that madness is not a natural, unchanging thing, but rather depends on the society in which it exists. He refers to assorted cultural, intellectual and economic structures which for him determine how madness is known and experienced within a given society. In this way, society constructs its experience of madness. The history of madness, maintains Foucault from 1961 onwards, cannot be an account of changing attitudes to a particular disease or state of being that remains constant as psychiatry would have it. Historically and across cultures, it is constructed and viewed differently, and the medical construction of madness as a mental disorder is merely one way of it being manufactured out of a multitude of possibilities.

Foucault claims in *Madness and Civilisation* that after the Renaissance (the arts and intellectual movements associated with the period between the fourteenth–seventeenth centuries) enormous houses of confinement were built in France. He argues that at the end of the Middle Ages there was general uneasiness in Europe about the mad living in the midst of communities. According to Foucault, 'ships of fools' had been used as an actual way of expelling mad people from the rest of the population to endlessly float along seas and canals. However, he believes that it also served as an allegory to represent fears about sin, evil and unreason within their midst and thereby quarantining the mad in the imagination.

One per cent of the population of Paris were eventually to be put in institutions such as the *Hôpital Général*. This one per cent was made-up of criminals, the idle, the poor and the insane. The reason for segregating the mad and other 'social deviants' from the rest of the population and from each other was not, postulates Foucault, primarily to do with a humanitarian concern by the authorities or because they were perceived to be in need of medical attention. Rather, it was so that these social deviants could be better controlled by the State. They served as an example of what was 'normal' and what was 'abnormal' so that the State could define clearly its power at a time when the economic structure of Europe was changing from clear-cut hierarchies and roles based on agriculture to a much more messy set of social relationships and a move towards industrial production. Those who were confined were classified as social deviants because they threatened to operate as a negative model with regard to what was required from the population – commitment to the needs of industry. To be lazy, impoverished or mad, was socially deviant because it was immoral. Morality had become defined by the Christian Church and the rising elites through work. Those who would not or could not work were construed as 'dangerous'. The mad were a dangerous class who would be (or were to be) controlled by those developing a new field of medicine – psychiatry.

Foucault is directly contradicting the history of psychiatry as progressive. For him, Esquirol was not a pioneer of valid insights and effective treatments from which the psychiatrists who followed him could learn from and build upon to the point where, at some as yet unreached point, madness would be comprehended completely and cured if not prevented. Psychiatry's history and predictions of steady advancement with the past scientific leaps (for example, the discovery of anti-psychotic and anti-depressant drugs) with further leaps pending (in particular the promised discovery of the gene or genes responsible for schizophrenia) is challengeable both in terms of the authenticity of these claims and their social worth.

For Foucault (1988), psychiatry helped resolve a paradox over the 'intelligibility' of criminal acts from the early part of the nineteenth century onwards. The growing commitment to rationalism and individualism, as a consequence of industrialisation, meant that the criminal justice system focused on the personal responsibility of the miscreant. Within this setting, a discourse of 'disclosure' is demanded. In what in effect becomes an undisclosed pact, psychiatrists offer their patients a way of abrogating personal responsibility for whatever has led them to seek medical help or led others to complain about them. During the interviewing of the patient, the psychiatrist's part of the pact is to avoid moral and judicial judgement and the patient's part is enacted by revealing his/her personal history, thoughts, behaviours and emotions. Supplying symptoms during this confessional removes fault.

By the nineteenth century, courts were interested in the criminal as well as the crime and the penalty. Judges, jurors and lawyers expected to be provided with details not only of the crime and the immediate circumstances but of the personal and social history of the accused. All-the-better if it was accompanied by a confession of madness or revelations which could be construed as a mental disorder. Moreover, unintelligible crime, where no motivating factors were disclosed by the accused or discovered by the court, is to be understood as not the responsibility of the perpetrator and thereby 'excusable' as an act of madness. Re-categorised as such, insane murders became the province of psychiatry. Trials of 'monstrous crimes' such as the killing of children for no apparent purpose allowed psychiatry to penetrate successfully the criminal justice system. Medical experts adjudicated over such crimes, justifying the legitimacy of their interventions by demonstrating that no 'reason' could be explicated.

Pierre Rivière's own power struggles are superimposed onto these social scenarios resulting in a morass of cause and effect connections. He is at war with himself, his family, community and society. His behaviours, verbal and written accounts are not consistent. They are indicative of a jumbled and embattled psyche. But Rivière, whether mad or bad, is not merely a person acting in a social vacuum, whose motives, actions and punishment can be located only at an individual level, as psychiatry and the criminal justice system, in the main, presume.

To recap, the Rivière case contributes to Foucault's position launched in *Madness and Civilisation* and other publications on the futility of attempting to expound on past events unless there is comprehensive knowledge about the social context in which those events took place. Even this contextualised knowledge may not, suggests Foucault, make 'knowing' indisputable. Further, Foucault maintains that facts about reality, in general, are always contingent upon standpoint and setting. Set alongside these viewpoints, Rivière for Foucault evinces the tenuousness of medical understanding of madness, as well as murder. A more recent case exemplifies well Foucault's contentions regarding the fragility of facts, the flakiness or reality and notably the fuzziness of psychiatric episteme.

Anders Breivik

On 22 July 2011, new agencies from across the world took notice of bombings in the capital of Norway, and shootings on Utøya Island some 25 miles from Oslo. Both of these events were found to have been instigated by a Norwegian citizen, Anders Breivik. In the subsequent days, months and years after these events, narratives were assembled by a host of journalists, the police, politicians and academics including myself. I was interviewed by the BBC some days after 22 July 2011 about my thoughts, such as they were at the time, on these events and to speculate about Breivik's mental state.

To begin with, the raw details of the bombings and shootings mutated across these and within these various narrations. Initially, there were few details of how many people had been injured and killed, figures were offered by the Norwegian police, but this was still being revised up and down days afterwards. It was first reported in some parts of the press that the perpetrator was thought to be a foreigner, and then more specifically supposed a Muslim immigrant. When the killer's identity was given as a white, blond, blue-eyed, middle-class Christian Norwegian with declared right-wing and anti-immigration views the earlier narratives which by then were converging on 'Islamic terrorism' had to be re-fashioned. Subsequently, opinions were garnered from members of the public, a plethora of experts, his friends, associates, and members of his family (including his father), about his childhood, whether or not he was part of a 'cell' or working alone, and of course about his motive. Further opinions were sought from these sources concerning whether or not he was mad or bad, and how much his badness or madness was caused by a fault in him or in his society, or perhaps in the wider, global society.

How Breivik's killings should be regarded legally and culturally in present and historical terms (for example, as domestic homicides or crimes against humanity) and how he should be dealt with also became key elements for debate. Moreover, concern was expressed in the media, by the public, professionals, and politicians about the effects on the social structure and culture of a society based on liberal democratic value, and on how best to mourn and commemorate the victims at both the personal and political levels.[2]

The available narratives to support innumerable stories were, therefore, plentiful, and they continue. More recent headlines from the news media include:

Norwegian mass murderer Anders Breivik's father to publish book: Jens Breivik's My Fault? A Father's story will deal with his role in life of killer and is said to be 'self-trial' by ex-diplomat.

The Guardian, *August 2014*

Breivik bomb van exhibited on Norway massacre anniversary.

Reuters Canada, 2015

Furthermore, as with Rivière, a document was written by the perpetrator. This is a political 'manifesto' rather than a personal memoir, and it was compiled prior to his killings rather than afterwards as Rivière had done. In his manifesto, Breivik indicates his preparedness for killings which he then made openly available on the Internet.[3] Moreover, Breivik's conduct and motivation have inspired a stage-play as had Rivière's. This stage-play bestows an interpretation which could have been inspired by Foucault because it adopts his sociological manner of exploring the contexts and constructions surrounding Breivik (Walker, 2013).

Extracts quoted below from the British *The Independent* newspaper printed the week after the killings with the title 'What turned Anders Breivik into Norway's worst nightmare?' highlight myriad of intricacies and inconsistencies in the search for a commanding narrative. By then what he did had been agreed: 77 people killed and 242 injured when he bombed government buildings in Oslo and subsequently shot young Labour Party supporters staying at an island camp. What had not been agreed – and still is not agreed – are the reasons. The article refers to how Breivik was being labelled in the media as a 'monster' and an 'obsessive'. Other more formalised ideas were posed:

> Some [psycho]analysts … advance the theory that Breivik had deep feelings of sexual inadequacy … [H]e subconsciously sought compensation through gross acts of violence carried out with the help of an assortment of obviously 'phallic' weapons … Political commentators … say that consensus politics conducted Norwegian-style have resulted in a form of extreme egalitarianism.
>
> *Paterson and Taylor, 2011*

Was he to be regarded as a monster, an obsessive, and/or sexually inadequate? On the other hand was the renowned fairness of Norwegian society somehow responsible for squashing his personality and needs, and thereby inducing such extreme compensatory actions in a similar way to how Foucault's colleagues Peter and Favret argue that Rivière's lethal deeds were shaped by an unfair French social system?

As with Rivière, with Breivik, there was no disagreement about who had carried out the killings. As with Rivière there were equivocations from within the medical profession regarding Breivik's madness or badness, and these are illustrated in the following extract taken from a BBC news item referring to the trial in 2012:

> A string of forensic and prison psychiatrists have told this court they think Breivik is not psychotic and therefore accountable ... Before the trial, psychiatrists commissioned by the court had found Breivik insane, suffering from paranoid schizophrenia, and therefore not responsible for his actions.
>
> *BBC News, 2012b*

Amidst medical equivocality about Breivik's sanity, the Norwegian prosecutor accepted that he should be placed in a secure psychiatric facility rather than prison. Breivik insisted in court that he was sane, and had a justifiable reason for conducting the bombings and shootings, that is to stop the 'Islamification' of Norway if not Western Europe. He and his lawyers, therefore, argued that he should be sent to prison, not to a mental hospital. For Breivik, it was rational to kill governmental workers and these young supporters of a party which was, in his view, supporting lax controls over immigration into Norway especially of those people adhering to Islam.

Contributing to the discord over Breivik's mental state, trial Judge Wenche Arntzen stated that he suffered from 'narcissistic personality characteristics' but was not psychotic (Arntzen quoted in BBC News, 2012). She then sentenced Breivik to a minimum of 10 years and a maximum of 21 years in prison after the jury found him sane and therefore guilty.

Discussing it better

Foucault was interviewed about *I, Pierre Rivière, having slaughtered my mother, my sister, and my brother...* one year after it was published (Lotringer, 1996). In the interview, he explains why he and his team had decided to decipher the meaning of the documented performances and the contiguous occurrences in what he refers to as 'this magnificent case'. Rivière's killings had occurred – points out Foucault in the interview – at a time when the discourse of the 'shrinks' (who for him are psychiatrists, psychologists, psychoanalysts, and criminologists) was igniting. His highlighting of the case, some 150 years later, was, he explained to the interviewer, intended to provoke twentieth-century shrinks into 'discussing it better' than had, in his view, their nineteenth-century colleagues. As he didn't think they were capable of such shrewdness, this would, he discloses, afford him the opportunity to reprise his intellectual attack on the legitimacy of the medical (psychiatric) discourse with regard to madness.

Ingrid Melle (2013), Professor of Psychiatry at the University of Oslo, has published an article titled 'The Breivik Case and what Psychiatrists can Learn from it' in the journal of the World Psychiatric Association. She comments in this article that the imprecision of Breivik's diagnosis may be down to the combined factors of differences in when the different assessments of his mental state were made, and confusion over the two main classification systems. She also posits that diagnostic criteria should not be taken as 'rules of law' but rather 'pragmatic definitions'. The 'magnificent case' of Breivik, therefore, exposes continuing contention over psychiatric diagnosis, and as Melle hints, 'the shrinks' still need to be provoked into 'discussing it better'.

Personal history

Foucault in the interview mentioned above questions a mainstay in the practice of psychiatry. To justify a diagnosis of madness the patients' personal history, and in particular, his mental background is explored. That is, there is retrospective searching for abnormalities from childhood onwards, and perhaps also in the personal history of members of his/her family. Elements of the patient's past performance are converted into abnormal signs and symptoms to justify a diagnosis.

With Rivière the range of 'mental maladies' for the neophyte French psychiatrists to choose from was relatively limited and in the end focused on one (monomania). With Breivik, Norwegian psychiatrists can choose one or more from the hundreds contained in the two main mental disorder classification systems, including many alternative personality disorders apart from that of the narcissistic. This may, as Melle (2013) points out, may be more a hindrance than a help in the process of psychiatric assessment.

There were approximately a score of verbal and documented details of Rivière's personal history made available for medical practitioners, legal officials and later Foucault, to peruse. However, there is a flood of information about Breivik's upbringing and personal habits and relationships for both the professional and amateur to peruse not only on the internet but in books many of which are attributed as authoritative, definitive or vital.

One such publication, written by Norwegian journalist Aage Borchgrevink (2012), attempts to link the Breivik's childhood experiences to the content of his manifesto. Another example is a book written by another Norwegian journalist, Åsne Seierstad (2015). Seierstad also offers detailed descriptions of Breivik's childhood and in particular his relationship with his mother, to try to explain why this sane person, as his mother believes him to be, comes to hold such crazy ideas – the ones that lead him to mass murder.

An example, however, of a purported authoritative account which steers away from the minutiae of personal history, is that provided by Norwegian social anthropologist Sindre Bangstad (2014). He contends that the political mainstreaming of racist ideologies throughout Europe gave licence to Breivik's actions. This thesis chimes with the view of Peter and Favret (see above) regarding the root social rather than individual reasons for such outbursts of violence.

The pioneers of the mental division of medicine in the nineteenth century, having begun to formalise and extend their practice into the courts were now in the business of not only separating madness from normality but unravelling madness from badness. By the time Breivik was in court, psychiatry had succeeded in installing itself as one, if not the, most called upon discipline of expert witnessing in criminal law as well as an inherent part of mental health and mental capacity tribunals (Rix, 2011).

Foucault observes that Pierre Rivière's personal history was used by those medical practitioners who believed he was mad as core evidence to support their new legal position. His propensity for crucifying animals and scaring other children was indicative, they argued, of eventual murderous madness. Breivik reportedly had difficult family relationships during his childhood (his parents divorced when he was very young), particularly with his mother, and was somewhat rebellious as an adolescent (Seierstad, 2015).

Crucifying animals and scaring other children may be unusual if indulged regularly and with heightened cruelty and veracity. To have a good relationship with one's parents and teachers is patently preferable to perpetually quarrelling with them. However, to classify all those who had been somewhat less than careful with their pets, who have frightened one of their siblings or peers, or who had in childhood disagreed with parents and didn't do as instructed by a teacher, as mad and possibly criminally insane, would certainly need a vast increase in the number of psychiatrists to deal with them. Such an expansion in numbers and narrative would lead to the broadening of the discourse of psychiatry, and increase the power of psychiatry.

For Foucault, this growth in the power of psychiatry had begun in the age of the 'Great Confinement', and was intensifying at the time of Rivière. Furthermore, for Foucault, it is not only the profession of medicine which had created a powerful speciality but it has been joined – often fractiously and sometimes in direct competition – by other types of 'shrinks'. He is particularly exercised by psychoanalysts.

Sigmund Freud

Foucault (Lotringer, 1996) had, he claims, set out in his and his colleagues' book on Rivière to provoke the 'shrinks' into discussing better their idea of madness. One such 'shrink' (and there was only one according to Foucault) who did take up his challenge to better discuss madness was dealt by him dismissively:

> [T]hey were literally reduced to silence: not a single one spoke up and said: 'Here is what Rivière was in reality. And I can tell you now what couldn't be said in the 19th century.' Except for one fool, a psychoanalyst … With this exception no one had anything to say.
>
> *Foucault, 1976, in Lotringer, 1996*

Despite much searching, I could not find Foucault's 'fool'. However, what I did find is a much more recent example of what Foucault might have regarded as a foolish analysis of Rivière by a Canadian psychoanalyst, Janet Oakes. On her website, Oakes presents a Freudian account of Rivière as well those of characters from the fictional work of playwrights William Shakespeare and Henrik Ibsen.

She applies a series of Freudian concepts, such as the 'Oedipus Complex' and 'castration anxiety':

> [Rivière's] unconscious Oedipal wishes toward his mother were contaminated by his fear of her destructive hostility … His mother's ongoing destructive attacks on his father and rejection of Pierre cause him to fear castration more from her than from his father.
>
> *Oakes, 2006*

Oakes elaborates on how Rivière had a fear of becoming ensnared into having sexual intimacy with females of any sort including his grandmothers, his sisters and even hens. The conflict between this sexual fear and his natural sexual needs, for Oakes, generated in him the ego defence mechanism of 'reaction formation'. That is, unconsciously Rivière became intensely loyal and over-identified with his father to protect himself from consciously conceding his hostility towards him (his father). The underlying enmity from a son directed towards his father, for Freud, is a consequence of the former becoming a rival for mothers' sexual attention. It is also the consequence, for Freud, of son's fear that the father's potential reaction to his sexual prospecting may be to castrate him. For Freud, the Oedipus Complex and Castration Anxiety are normal phases of childhood development. But, argues Oakes, in Rivière they had remained unresolved and caused what she describes as 'psychic pressure', which then led him to kill his mother, brother and sister.

Much of Oakes's extolling about Rivière is probably impenetrable and bizarre to those who have not studied deeply Freud's multifarious and entwined concepts. The following are the basics of Freud's outlook on the human mind which relate to what Oakes appears to be applying to Rivière.

Eroticism and aggression

Humans, Freud argued, are fundamentally driven by their innate aggressive and erotic desires (Freud original 1920, in Strachey, 2001). The human mind, Freud proposed, contains three abstract structures (Freud, original 1923, in Strachey, 2001). These are:

> (a) the id: this is the primitive drive to find instant and on-going erotic pleasure using liberal amounts of aggression if necessary and without heed to the needs of others.
> (b) the ego: this is what the individual comes to appreciate as his/her real 'self', his/her conscious awareness of the world, memory and intellectual functioning.
> (c) the super-ego; this is the collection of moral standards handed down to the child from significant others (for example, parents, peers and teachers) and society at large; it is the conscience, and as such it, along with the ego, controls the primitive drives of the id.

Young children, Freud postulated, have sexual desire emanating from the id. At the age of between 3–5 years male children focus their desire unconsciously on their mother. This is the stage of Oedipus, named after a mythical Greek King who unintentionally murders his father and then marries a woman who turns out to be his mother. Later Freudians (specifically Carl Jung, 1970) formulated an equivalent for females which occurred at approximately the same age as males and their Oedipus Complex – the 'Electra Complex' – from another Greek myth in which there is unconscious sexual desire aimed at the father (Electra's father was also the King). This they do on the discovery that they do not have a penis and blame their mother for this inadequacy (boys at this point are worrying about being castrated by their father). They then turn their sexual attention towards their father whom they envy for having what they haven't got – a penis. The ego and eventually the super-ego need to resolve the Complexes.

However, even the uninitiated in the verbiage and visions of the psychoanalysts will pick up that Oakes believes there was a lot of sex and violence going on in Rivière's (unconscious) mind long before he killed anyone. Freud, however, thought there was a lot of both going on in everyone's mind. If anything goes wrong in anyone's childhood with the development of the mind's structures and their interrelationships, or with the normal resolution to the Oedipal impulse, then assorted types of badness or madness can be the result, which may require years of psychoanalysis to repair.

Freud's legacy

Freudian notions are commonplace in Western thought long after the death of their creator, and some are widely accepted as having veracity (for example, the role of the unconscious in human thinking, behaviour and emotions: Western, 1998). Breivik has been scrutinised psychoanalytically (in the second-hand sense) by psychoanalysts, one of whom is Siri Gullestad, Professor of Clinical Psychology at the University of Oslo. Gullestad is a practising psychoanalyst and member of the International Psychoanalytic Association, referring to Breivik he states:

> In this [psychoanalytic explanation] ideologies are interpreted in a dialectical movement, both through a 'hermeneutics of suspicion' … with a view to grasp psychological causes, and in a 'teleological' frame … with a view to the values and intentions that the individual identifies with.
> *Gullestad, 2013*

Many of Freud's opinions have come to be held as foolish by followers of other branches of psychology, psychotherapy and psychiatry. Feminists have been incensed, quite understandably, by such notions that women are unavoidably envious of men having a penis and are not quite human because they are not men (Horney, 1993; Greer, 1970). As a consequence, Freud's ideas have been modified, some drastically, by post-Freud analysts, particularly those who describe themselves as psychodynamic rather than psychoanalytic therapists (Western, 1998). Although Freud was medically trained, he believed madness to be a real entity and considered himself to be a scientist. However, those who today avow scientific explanations and remedies (particularly those psychiatrists who are steeped in the neurology and cognitive-behavioural therapists) are especially critical, decrying his lack of verifiable evidence for his ideas (Leahy, 2011; Esterson, 2015).

What Freud did do for the study of the mind and human performance generally was not only to offer insights into how humans operate at an intra-psychic level but how there is an interaction between the individual and society (Bocock, 2002). Freud's sociological credentials emanate through his acknowledgement that there is for Freud always a tension between the needs of society and the drives of the individual (Freud original 1930, in Strachey, 2001). The personal compulsions of sex and violence are modified by society. The mind is susceptible to socialisation, but conformity does not bring complete contentment because of the individualistic-societal strain.

Ship of fools

Who really is the fool? Is the fool Freud or Foucault, or perhaps Esquirol? Certainly, Freud is justifiably accused of making sweeping assumptions from his limited sample of patients who had already experienced psychological problems. However, Foucault is certainly suspect as a historian. He tends to be selective in which events and cases he uses to support his ideas. That is so with Pierre Rivière. From this one case, he and his colleagues assert connections between the deaths of three people killed by this peasant from an otherwise obscure village to the whole of the nineteenth-century French social system and the beginnings of the power of psychiatry. Furthermore, they use that one case to foment the proposition that madness, rather than being a real disorder has been contrived by powerful groups to seem as such.

The frail foundation of Foucault's historical data, and the foolishness of his scholarship is addressed by sociologist Andrew Scull (of whom more will be found in Chapter 2). Scull (2011) accuses Foucault of employing a 'one-eyed lens' to look at the history of madness. Foucault's academic work on the history of madness and mad-doctoring argues Scull, is seductive but superficial, relying on dubious and dated references. He remarks that Foucault was inventive but rather than this being a compliment regarding the originality of his ideas it is meant as a criticism. That is, Scull is suggesting that Foucault either misinterpreted or invented facts to support his interesting intellectual compositions.

Scull (2007a) refers to Foucault's mistaken account in relation to the 'sightseeing' at the Bedlam madhouse in London. Foucault, points out Scull, asserts that a House of Commons Enquiry into conditions in England's madhouses during the period 1815–1816 had reported that the public could pay a penny on a Sunday to view the inmates of Bethlem Hospital (Bedlam) and that nearly 100,000 such viewings happened annually. However, Scull contends that the Enquiry did not mention this profitable form of mass voyeurism in its report. This, for Scull, is not surprising as these viewings had been stopped in 1770 by the governors of Bethlem Hospital. Moreover, that there was a fixed fee of a penny or any other amount, suggests Scull, was likely to have been a fiction.

The notion espoused by Foucault of a 'Great Confinement' of the mad across Europe, including France, in the seventeenth and eighteenth centuries is for Scull, also mythical. It certainly did not occur in England until the nineteenth century:

> Vast museums of madness did not emerge until the nineteenth century (when they were purpose-built using taxpayers' funds).
>
> *Scull, 2007a, p.3*

Not only was there not a Great Confinement at the time stated by Foucault but most of those madhouses that did exist then had low numbers of inmates. Moreover, the reason given by Foucault for this Great Confinement, that madness disturbed the moral order, is mistaken. Why should there be in the seventeenth century, asks Scull, a sudden 'social sensibility' to the mad being in the community which then led to their mass confinement? Why should there be a radical break from thousands of years of mad people having lived amongst their families or having been free to wander where they wished (Scull, 2011)? Furthermore, points out Scull, Foucault's 'ships of fools' did not exist (Scull, 2007a), although this is somewhat unfair to Foucault as he had recognised that this was more of a metaphor than an actuality.

How do Esquirol's ideas about madness compare with those of Foucault? Who is more convincing? In a career working with the mad for 40 years, Esquirol recorded systematically what he observed and what sense could be made from those observations. He collected these observations by going out into the field. That is, on more than one occasion he travelled around France to see for himself how the mad were (not being) cared for, and from these observations judged what practically could be recommended to improve both the understanding of madness and the lot of the mad. Foucault's evidence tended to be obtained from the observations and publications of others mixed with his own ideas.

What did Foucault recommend as the alternative to the medical knowledge and medical vested 'intrusion' of physicians in the arena of madness? Foucault's intellectual innovativeness regarding madness is unsurpassed, but he doesn't offer much of any practical use.

To compare Foucault with Esquirol is perhaps unreasonable. The former was (only) a thinker whereas the latter both thought and acted on his thoughts. That said, Foucault's impractical thoughts have been and still are applied to many areas of medical, health and social care practice (Peterson and Bunton, 2012).

In particular, they have become standard contemplative fulcra of non-standard practice in psychiatry and psychiatric nursing, psychology, and psychotherapy (Roberts, 2005; Hook, 2010; Besley, 2002). Moreover, the psychiatric science of Esquirol is suspect. Specifically, his foremost category of madness, that is monomania, was considered not long after his death (and at times during his life) to be without scientific foundation (Huertas, 2008).

Was Foucault not foolish but mad? Foucault was fascinated by the link between extreme sexual practices and extreme sado-masochism which he believed could offer novel and creative ways gaining intense pleasure. Foucault saw liberation from social constraints that dictated parameters to thought, knowledge and behaviour, by engaging in what he described as 'suicidal orgies'. For Foucault, ultimate pleasure and freedom are inexorably coupled with death (Miller, 1993). It was the freedom to indulge in unregulated (homosexual) erotic pleasure because of, not despite, the risks, that led directly to his own demise. For Foucault, the ultimate control over living was gained by not being scared of dying. In his biographical analysis of Foucault, James Miller recorded Foucault's response, whilst he was lecturing at the University of California in 1983, to an undergraduate student's question about personal autonomy:

> Who could be scared of AIDs? You could be hit by a car tomorrow. Even crossing the street was dangerous! If sex with a boy gives me pleasure – why renounce such pleasure? We have the power … we shouldn't give it up.
>
> *Foucault in Miller, 1993, p.353*

Foucault died the following year.

Summary

Michel Foucault used the nineteenth-century case of Pierre Rivière to highlight his idea that reality and truth are sold as such by the powerful but countless other realities and truths are possible. Knowledge, therefore, is always disputable. In particular, he contests the knowledge espoused by scientifically-orientated psychiatrists from Jean-Etienne Esquirol and Wilhelm Griesinger onwards that madness is a real and comprehensible disorder (or multiplicity of disorders) akin to physical disorder.

Implicitly and at times explicitly Foucault denigrates the 'shrinks' who do not accept that madness is manufactured – describing one as a fool. However, today, across the world, the shrinks in the form of psychiatrists are either in charge or are making great strides to take charge of how madness should be understood and managed. That is psychiatry's idea of madness dominates. But as the twenty-first-century case of Anders Breivik indicates, that domination is built on an idea which is – so far – far from concrete.

However, original shrinks Esquirol and Griesinger, although perhaps foolishly seeking *the* truth about the workings of mind – and in particular the mind's bond with the brain – were very much aware that many forms of madness have complex aetiologies and that frequently there is interplay between predisposing and precipitating factors found both within the individual and society. Hence, they cannot be accused of biological-reductionism. That is, they did not reduce all normal and abnormal human performance to the urges of biology, an accusation frequently levelled at psychiatry as it became more absorbed with the minutiae of the performance of the brain, by both members of its own profession (Tallis, 2004, 2014), and, more frequently, by sociologists including Scull:

> So far as psychiatry is concerned, we once again live in an era where simplistic and biologically reductionist accounts of mental disorder enjoy widespread currency. Patients and their families have learned to attribute their travails to biochemical abnormalities, to faulty neurotransmitters, and to genetic defects.
>
> *Scull, 2005a*

Esquirol and Griesinger also understood that their knowledge about cerebral function and malfunction would in all probability be superseded if not contradicted as the science of madness progressed. Furthermore, although Esquirol and Griesinger were authoritarian, they were also humanitarian. They promoted vigorously their ideas about madness and endorsed enthusiastically psychiatry as the most important specialism in the madness arena, but they were also engaged with the everyday suffering of their patients and attempted to do well by them. That they occupied ivory-towers did not divorce them from what may have been a manufactured reality but one that was experienced as real by those affected by and those dealing with madness.

Notes

1 There is a long-standing discussion about the differences and similarities between psychopathy and anti-social-behaviour disorder as well as sociopathy, dissocial personality disorder and dangerous and severe personality disorder. In the academic, clinical, and popular forensic literature they are used as synonyms, overlapping types, or as distinctive categories (Hare, 1996; MacKenzie, 2014; Verona, and Patrick (2015). Lack of remorse, however, tends to be common to all of these classifications. I will for the main part use psychopathy as common for these other identifiers.

2 I have not listed the media reports on Breivik mentioned in this and the preceding paragraph as most remain in the public domain and are easily accessible via electronic search systems of news-agencies and newspapers such as the BBC, Reuters, *The Guardian* and CNN.

3 I avoid referencing Breivik's Manifesto in what is probably a futile attempt not to encourage the propagation of the ideas contained within.

Further reading

Esquirol, E. (1845) (translated from original French edition by Hunt E) *Mental Maladies: Treatise on Insanity*. Philadelphia: Lea and Blanchard.

Foucault, M. (1975) (editor) *I, Pierre Riviere, Having Slaughtered My Mother, My Sister and My Brother: A Case of Parricide in the 19th Century*. New York: Pantheon.

Foucault, M. (1971) *Madness and Civilization: A History of Insanity in the Age of Reason*. London: Tavistock.

2

INCARCERATION AND CONTROL

John Perceval

British Prime Minister Spencer Perceval was shot dead on 11 May 1812. It is questionable as to how much of a loss his death was to the country overall, but certain groups towards whom he had targeted his political chagrin during his three years as Prime Minister, would not have been dismayed. These included: Catholics; the Irish; Napoleon; the press; gamblers; adulterers; boozers; hunters; and slavers. His murderer, John Bellingham, did not represent any of these groups. He had his own reason for despising Perceval (Hanrahan, 2012).

Bellingham had twice been imprisoned in Russia, the first time over an alleged financial misdemeanour, and the second time for complaining to the Russian authorities about the reason for the first imprisonment. By the time of his release he was impoverished, and on returning to England he petitioned the British Government for compensation regarding both his present financial position and his past imprisonment. Bellingham's assassination of the Prime Minister by his own admission was the consequence of him bearing a grudge for the Government's lack of concern over his situation and in particular towards Prime Minister Perceval for not intervening on his behalf:

> If they [the British Government] had listened to my case this court would not have been engaged in this case, but Mr. Perceval obstinately refusing to sanction my claim in Parliament I was driven to despair, and under these agonizing feelings I was impelled to that desperate alternative which I unfortunately adopted.
>
> *Bellingham, quoted in Proceedings of the Old Bailey, 1812*

His despair, agony, and desperation may not have been assuaged by killing the Prime Minister given that he was hanged and his body dissected for medical research (Proceedings of the Old Bailey, 1812). The loss to Prime Minister Perceval's wife and offspring was assuaged by a substantial indemnity from the government (Linklater, 2013).

The improvement in the financial circumstances of the dead Prime Minister's family meant that when one of the 12 children, John, became by his own admission insane he was placed – against his will – in prestigious, expensive and purportedly humane asylums. After his eventual discharge, John Perceval was able to spend some of the family's Government-donated wealth to support himself with his writing projects. Specifically, he was able to spend time authoring an incredibly insightful two-volume text about his experience in asylums and about the nature of his madness and madness in general. The first of these texts was produced in 1838 and the second in 1840. The latter was to come with an expansive title:

> *A Narrative of the treatment experienced by a Gentleman during a state of mental derangement; Designed to explain the causes and the nature of insanity, and to expose the injudicious conduct pursued towards many unfortunate sufferers under that calamity, by John Perceval Esq.*

Usually, however, the combined text is referred to as *Perceval's Narrative* although there are various titles and subtitles used in the many edited versions that have been published since the original. The one I am using in this chapter was re-published in 1962 and titled concisely as *Perceval's Narrative: A Patient's Account of His Psychosis 1830–1832*. This edition was compiled by biologist, linguist, psychotherapist and anthropologist Gregory Bateson (he was married to the renowned anthropologist Margaret Mead). More is said of Bateson below.

Brislington Asylum

The first asylum in which Perceval was compulsorily placed was an expensive private institution at Brislington near Bristol, England. Buildings within a large rural estate had been bought in 1799 by physician, surgeon and Quaker, Edward Long Fox (Smith, 1999). These buildings and surrounding land formed the original asylum which opened in 1804. A series of detached houses were later joined into one large building, an architecturally and psychologically imposing centrepiece. Such power-laden centrepieces were replicated in many institutions for the mad (Morrall and Hazelton, 2000).

However, the regime at the Brislington Asylum (which became known locally as 'Brislington House') expressly espoused a humane philosophy. Moreover, it catered for a cross-section of social classes, including the nobility, although each was segregated from the other. Edward Long Fox died in 1929 and its ownership was inherited by his two sons, one of whom, Francis, took over its management and against whom Perceval was to fulminate. Despite Fox's declared commitment to compassion, Perceval was to accuse his incarcerators of inhumanity towards him and his fellow inmates (Bateson, 1962).

What had led to the incarceration of Perceval? According to Bateson's commentary, Perceval's childhood and adolescence were conventional. His early adulthood also seems to have been ordinary for his family's social rank. He worked first a private tutor and then enlisted as an army officer. In 1830 at the age of 27 he entered Oxford University. However, he didn't last long at Oxford. During his time in the military, he had become troubled by his religious beliefs, which he had absorbed from his father. Perceval went off to Scotland to visit an extreme evangelistic cult. This cult advocated a communication technique aimed at spiritual enlightenment which entailed 'speaking in tongues'. Psychiatry dubs speaking in tongues as 'glossolalia', which may be interpreted as a sign of mental disorder (Koić et al., 2005). Notwithstanding their own vulnerability to a psychiatric diagnosis, to the cult members Perceval appeared to be too unstable mentally to remain in their midst.

Having fallen out with the Scottish cultists, Perceval went off to Dublin where he became involved with a prostitute. Perceval became concerned that he may have contracted syphilis. This was not an unusual worry given the high prevalence of both prostitutes and venereal disease in Ireland at that time (Ward, 2010). When the supposed symptoms of syphilis dissipated, Perceval claimed that his sexual healing had been due to God's intervention rather than through the medication he had been prescribed. His claim has some cogency as he did believe in the existence of God, and there were no truly effective cures for syphilis if that is what he had contracted, until the discovery of antibiotics in the mid-twentieth century (Ward, 2012). Moreover, he had apparently only taken half the prescribed medicine (Bateson, 1962).

Perceval's physical ill-health, imagined or real, had resolved but his mental state became more erratic to the point that he had to be physically restrained in his Dublin lodgings. His family was informed of his situation, and in December of 1830 his oldest brother came to take him from Dublin back to England. The journey on the boat across the Irish Sea proved to be eventful.

On board the boat Perceval in his *Narrative* refers to his 'wildest delusions' which he admits put all those on board in peril. His delusions centre upon him needing to be thrown overboard as a penance for his sins and so that the crew would be saved. His attempt to go overboard led to a violent rumpus between him and his 'servant', a man hired by his brother to help escort him back to England:

> My servant struggled with me, and could only get me down by lying on me … At last, he got a pair of steel handcuffs on me … I struck at him with my manacled arms, endeavouring to kill him.
>
> *Perceval in Bateson, 1962, p.57*

Having done battle with his servant and lost, he declares that his mind became more settled and that he was pleased to note that as they advanced on their destination of Bristol, the crew was still alive. But his skirmishing with others turns inward:

> My mind was recovering from the shock of its horrid delusions... At the
> same time I felt an indignant hate towards the voices that had so acutely
> terrified me.
>
> *Perceval in Bateson, 1962, p.57*

This conflict between his needing to obey these intrusive thoughts and resisting
their instructions continues for much of his madness years.

At this point no-one, not the cultists, the boats' crew, Perceval's brother and
the rest of his family, nor Perceval, was offering an alternative understanding
for what his performance implied: all agreed he was insane. For Perceval's
family, to have one of its members deemed mad was likely to have been highly
stigmatising given their high social status, and which therefore may well have
been in itself a good enough excuse to seek incarceration for him. This was
not an uncommon tactic for the upper and middle classes and was relatively
easily achieved, as long as it could be afforded, because privately-run madhouses
had become much more widely available. The nineteenth century also heralded
the mass movement of the mad into publically-run asylums which could then
accommodate large numbers of the lower classes deemed to be suffering from
some sort of mental infirmity whether this was insanity, idiocy, or epilepsy
(Porter, 1987).

Keepers and attendants

By early January of 1831, Perceval found himself in the Fox family's asylum and
in the company of an interesting assortment of lunatics and their custodians,
the keepers and attendants. The early private and subsequent public madhouses
needed only keepers and attendants to contain their charges rather than to
offer compassionate nurturing let alone any form of fruitful alleviation of
madness (Nolan, 1993). From about 1830 onwards there was a proliferation
in the number of institutions for the mad and a substantiation of their medical
management. At this point male keepers were to become attendants and female
keepers became nurses, thereby denoting a modicum of care expected in the
delivery of their role rather than pure control. Psychiatric nursing was to emerge
as a formal occupational pursuit once the medical profession had thoroughly
gained governance over the trade in madness towards the later part of the
nineteenth century.

The keepers and also the attendants, whilst at liberty to dole out discipline,
were anything but disciplined. They were generally from the very lowest section
of society, unskilled and untrained, feckless and/or alcoholic. Some were ex-
patients. They were selected from these social strata because they were cheap
to engage in the service of the asylum managers. There also was a need for a
complement of males to be employed mainly for their brute strength to man-
handle uncooperative or frenzied inmates especially when unpopular treatments
were to be administered (Scull, 1979; Mellett, 1982).

However, the perception that the keepers and attendants were the lowest of the low in terms of proficiency and benevolence is considered by historian Leonard Smith (1988), to be an unjust generalisation. His argument is that given the values and conditions of the time, some of those attending to the mad were not unduly pitiless or without skills which could be either interpersonal or practical. Those with practical skills might be asked to help maintain the infrastructure (the asylum buildings needed to be looked after as well as their inhabitants) and to handle the everyday necessities of the institution (for example, preparing food and dealing with laundry). Moreover, given the potential and actual performance of some of their attendees, the conditions in which they worked, and the nature of the treatments ordered by their medical masters, I suggest that many were remarkably tolerant and compassionate including some of Perceval's overseers.

Perceval's descriptions of the 'lunatic doctors', their enforcers, and his fellow inmates (not all of whom were detained against their will) reveal specifics of pitifulness, harshness, but also kindliness. The personality of each with whom he has to share time and space in the two asylums in which he was placed is portrayed by him with the acumen of an accomplished novelist revealing the nuances of the story's characters. Each character in *Perceval's Narrative* is given a nickname. His relationship with several other inmates is described in detail, with specific attention to their mental misfortunes. Regarding his 'lunatic doctors' as he refers to the asylums' medical practitioners he is scathing, claiming that they were habitually harsh and ill-informed charlatans who concentrated on trying to control rather than to cure him. He did, however, have an ambivalent relationship with and variable attitudes towards his attendants, and they according to Perceval were similarly inconsistent towards him.

Perceval also explains how he attempted to manipulate his minders, at times to attempt to maintain his individuality and at other times merely to annoy them. When he lost these interpersonal power games there were regularly retributive consequences for him such as blows, restraint and seclusion.

Everyday life

Alongside the descriptions of staff and patients in Brislington there is detail in *Perceval's Narrative* of the sheer banality of everyday life in an asylum. He records the pattern of nearly every day which would begin with him being taken from his room to breakfast by an attendant between half-past six and seven o'clock. He would be seated in what he calls his 'niche' and strapped in place. Breakfast would be served at eight o'clock:

> My tea was placed before me … in a slop basin, on a small deal table, with a plate of bread and butter. And usually one hand was loosened from the straight waistcoat; at times I was fed by the hand.
>
> *Perceval in Bateson, 1962, p.75*

If the weather allowed, the patients would be escorted outdoors by the attendants for a walk lasting about one hour in the morning and afternoon. If not out walking, then Perceval remained tied in his niche. Lunch was served at one o'clock and tea (that is dinner) at seven o'clock after which the patients either made their own way to bed or were taken there by an attendant. Breaking-up this routine during the day was the occasional shave or bath. The diet afforded to Perceval, and presumably all the patients, was also routinised as well as undemanding for the palate. This consisted mainly of bread with butter, tea with milk, small amounts of beer and the intermittent provision of a pudding.

Perceval describes his surroundings in a more positive tone than he does his routine and diet:

> Dr. F.'s madhouse stood in a very fine and picturesque country, and near a steep and wooded bank that bordered the river. At one elevated spot that commanded a view down the valley, a natural or artificial precipice yawned in the red soil, crowned with a small parapet.
>
> *Perceval in Bateson, 1962, p.116*

It is to be remembered that Brislington House was regarded as a prestigious private asylum and its prestige was in no small part due to the quality of the physical environment. However, most of the new wave of public asylums in the nineteenth century did have pleasant external surroundings as they were deliberately built on the outside of towns in rural areas.

The tedium of the daily schedules would only alter, sometimes dramatically so, when violence erupted, or when a patient was considered non-violent enough to take tea with Dr. Fox and his family and thereby removed for a few hours into a more salubrious setting than what Perceval reports to be the noisy and crowded common room in which most of a patients' day was spent. During an unspecified number of times towards the end of his stay in Brislington Perceval took tea with the Foxes. Although not violent, he mentions that he was still hallucinating, with voices telling him how to behave (for example, not to drink the wine he was offered). He did, however, seem well enough to refer to the beauty of the female servant who attended those meals and had a similar appreciation for Dr Fox's wife who, without explanation, he nicknames 'Repentance' (Perceval in Bateson, 1962).

Erving Goffman

The monotonous routines and strict regulations of everyday life in the asylums have been investigated by the sociologist Erving Goffman (1922–1982). Canadian-born Goffman became one of the best-known sociologists of the twentieth century, introducing a range of thoughts into social science which have persisted into the twenty-first century (Jacobsen and Kristiansen, 2014).

Total institutions

Goffman's (1961) research into asylums consisted of outwardly working as a junior employee of a federal mental hospital containing 7,000 patients, but with the connivance of senior management, covertly operating as a researcher. His participant observation lasted for a year during which time he collected copious notes on the specifics of life led by the patients.

From the data Goffman accumulated in this mental hospital, he maintained that mental hospitals generally and monasteries, nunneries, boarding schools, gaols, concentration camps, and military establishments, provided for – and in many circumstances enforced – all aspects of an individual's existence. Patients, monks, nuns, pupils, prisoners and soldiers, eat, sleep, work and socialise within their respective institution. These, therefore, were for Goffman 'total institutions'.

The effects of living in a total institution argued Goffman, varied, but to a greater or lesser extent they led to institutionalisation. That is, the requirements of the institution, or at least the interests of those in charge, superseded the needs and norms of the individual. For example, nuns are obligated to follow the convent's tacit regime of supplication and contemplation, and prisoners are compelled to adhere to the gaol's patent rules concerning clothing and orderly conduct. What Goffman observed was that mental patients were not necessarily coerced (although Perceval was) but became 'conditioned' by institutional conventions which were frequently unstated. This left them in a state of psychological and social enfeeblement. Unlike nuns or prisoners, a mental patient was largely unaware of his/her institutional habituation, and therefore unlikely to dissent and thereby retain some degree of individuality. They became depersonalised.

Life as drama

Another idea from Goffman (1959), taken from an earlier study into how 'the self' is presented in everyday life is that patients and staff are engaged in a drama (as are all humans when dealing with other humans) in which each has a role with related scripts that indicate how they should act in any given situation. These scripts, proposed Goffman, are malleable depending on how the actors interact with each and how symbolic are the verbal and non-verbal messages being transferred between these actors. That is, some communications are taken as more important and pertinent than others because of, for example, the social status of the persons involved. A consultant psychiatrist telling a patient that he/she has clinical depression is likely to be taken more seriously than a friend telling another friend that he/she is very miserable. On being diagnosed with a mental or physical disorder, the temptation is to follow the script of the role associated with that disorder if this is known. If it is not known then multiple messages may move the individual in that direction (for example, official leaflets given to patients or information gleaned from Internet sources detailing the process of their disorder).

However, Russell Barton (1959), Physician Superintendent at Severalls Hospital in Colchester, England, had already medicalised what Goffman was to describe as institutionalisation. Barton coined the term 'institutional neurosis'. However, Barton's intention was not to add to psychiatry's lengthy lexicon of mental disorders. He did believe in the fact of madness, unlike Goffman who lent towards the position of madness being socially constructed thereby giving support to 'de-institutionalisation' (that is, non-medical care in and by the community). What Barton recommended was a much more benevolent type of institutional care: contact by patients with the outside world should be encouraged by the staff of the institution; there should be an overall reduction of drug treatments, an increase in personal possessions, meaningful work offered to patients; and a change of attitude amongst the staff to prevent depersonalisation.

Furthermore, Goffman and Barton along with Perceval realised that the institutionalisation experienced within mental hospitals conditioned patients to perform the role of 'good patient' in the way expected by the staff otherwise they would not be considered eligible for discharge. That is, the normal illness trajectory had to be, after an initial period of uncooperativeness, one of settling down to the psychologically dulling and collectivist way of life in the institution. This life could, however, stimulate persistent defiance (with Perceval this was violent defiance) which would then be met with an intensification of control with such remedies for rebellion as restraint and seclusion.

Cow-shed and gothic nightmare

On one occasion in Brislington, Perceval was placed in an outhouse in solitary confinement (although he usually slept in his own room but with an attendant frequently present) and shackled seemingly as punishment. He describes the filthy condition of his combined seclusion and restraint and his complete disempowerment thus:

> There was a mattress of straw, and a pillow of straw, both stinking … I was then strapped down with a broad strap over my chest, and my right arm was manacled to a chain in the wall … I conceived myself in circumstances hopelessly beyond my control.
>
> *Perceval in Bateson, 1962, p.94*

But rather than wallowing in misery in his cow-shed cell, Perceval comments that he was happy. It was, he remarks, peaceful in the cow-shed, and in his aloneness he could obey the voices if they commanded him to shout or sing, and there this wouldn't lead to him being hit by the attendants.

The power enjoyed by the staff of these total institutions meant that the arbitrary enactment of solitary isolation and corporeal curbing could take place unobserved by the outside world. So could medical experimentation. Live eels to induce an electric shock as treatment for those deemed psychologically disturbed had been used in Greco-Roman civilisation. Electro-convulsive-therapy became its successor in the 1930s, reaching a peak of usage, mainly on women and commonly without informed or any form of consent, in the 1950s (Berrios, 1996). However, in Britain, 50,000 people in 1980 were still receiving electric shocks as a treatment for clinical depression (Pippard and Ellam, 1981). Trepanning (drilling or smashing a hole in the skull) was practised also in ancient times and was a precursor of the mid-twentieth-century fad for leucotomies and lobotomies (severing bits of brain tissue) aimed specifically at reducing violent behaviour. Tens of thousands of those treated by psychiatrists in the USA alone underwent a markedly imprecise surgical laceration to the frontal regions of the cerebral cortex, many of which were performed specifically to reduce violent behaviour (Arnold, 2008).

Henry Cotton (1876–1933) was an arch proponent of psychiatry as a medical specialism. He had studied under distinguished psychiatrists, Emil Kraepelin, Alois Alzheimer and Adolf Meyer. Kraepelin (1856–1926), along with Jean-Étienne-Dominique Esquirol and Wilhelm Griesinger (see Chapter 1) had a huge influence on the early development of psychiatry and on how it is conducted today. For Esquirol, Griesinger and Kraepelin, madness (certainly the major mental disorders) is caused by faulty biology. Therefore, for psychiatry to be seen as a scientific discipline it requires a standardised classification system which accords cause, symptoms and treatment to each disorder. Quantified causation, symptoms and classification preside as the core tenets of twenty-first-century psychiatric theory and practice.

Notwithstanding an intermediary period when the psychology of Freud and succeeding theories which also focused on the mind became popular, Kraepelin's ideas concerning neuro-pathology have much in common with biological research into causation and pharmacological treatments of the late-twentieth century onwards. It was, however, another pioneer of psychiatry, Swiss Eugen Bleuler (1857–1939), who came-up with the most long-lasting and recognised diagnostic tag for madness when he changed Kraepelin's term of 'dementia praecox' to that of schizophrenia. Alzhemier (1864–1915) correctly attributed pre-senile dementia to pathological changes in the cerebral cortex and therefore can be counted as giving legitimisation to the 'fault biology' stance regarding at least this form of madness. Meyer (1866–1950) was to become a president of the American Psychiatric Association, and is known for deviating from the pure biological approach to madness through his search for psychological and social causative factors.

Cotton's contribution to early twentieth-century psychiatry created what sociologist Andrew Scull (2005b) refers to as a 'gothic nightmare' as a handful of megalomaniacal medical practitioners experimented almost with little heed to ethical considerations on a vulnerable captive audience. Cotton is singled out by Scull for his heightened displays of self-importance and surgical ruthlessness when he worked at Trenton State Psychiatric Hospital in New Jersey, USA, where had become its medical director at 30 years of age. One of his neurological procedures was the injection of what he regarded as a 'magic bullet' serum. This arsenic compound was introduced into the cranial cavity of patients suffering from general paralysis of the insane (that is tertiary syphilis). Cotton conducted the operation with an electric drill, whilst his patients were wide-awake although thoughtfully he did apply local anaesthesia to the scalp prior to inserting the serum.

Hundreds of pre-frontal lobotomies later in the 1930s were conducted on mentally disordered patients by neurologist Walter Freeman, assisted by his long-term colleague James Watts. Early in the next decade Freeman, again with Watts, decided to implement a novel surgical method he had learned from experiments by European psychiatrists. This involved using an ice-pick and a small mallet to smash his way through the eye-sockets of his patients to get at the white matter of the brain, having first, thoughtfully, rendered them unconscious with electrical shocks (Scull, 2011). Freeman continued to ice-pick his private patients until the late 1960s. By this time he had performed thousands of trans-orbital leucotomies.

Cotton's enthusiastic surgical extracting and refashioning of teeth, tonsils, gall-bladders, colons, testicles and rectums, was eventually to get him discredited within his own profession. He is, however, credited for his more humane interventions such as relieving patients from physical restraints when he was medical director at Trenton, although he stopped conducting surgery only on retirement (Scull, 2005b). Freeman did become *persona non grata* in the public sector and did eventually split from his colleague Watts, apparently because the latter thought their surgery had become too savage. He was finally banned from surgery, but not from practising other forms of psychiatry (Scull, 2005b).

Freeman's nemesis was, however, to come only long after his death. This came in the form of an autobiography by one of his patients, Howard Dully.

Howard Dully

Dully has become a celebrated survivor of psychiatric excess. He was at the age of 12 lobotomised by Freeman.

His account of his lobotomy has been recounted in the international news media (see for example Gajilan, 2005; ABC, 2002) and in a documentary broadcast on the USA National Public Radio (NPR, 2005). He has also published the story of his lobotomy in a book he co-authored with writer and newspaper editor Charles Fleming (Dully and Fleming, 2008). The book's content is supported by Dully's own memories and information gleaned from discussions he had with members of his family and relatives of lobotomy patients from that era as well as those of Freeman. Remarkably, he was also able to access his own medical file written by Freeman.

The details of Dully's life referred to in this and the next few paragraphs are taken from his and Fleming's book. Dully was born in 1948, in California, his mother had died from cancer when he was young, and his father soon remarried. It was his step-mother who was instrumental in having him declared officially as psychologically troubled and troublesome which was her judgement of him. Step-son and step-mother had a difficult relationship. He found her too strict and emotionally abusive, and she regarded his aggression, defiance, stealing, and uncleanliness, unacceptable. He was physically chastised regularly by both step-mother and father. Dully admits that he was, both at home and at school, a trouble-maker.

It was Dully's step-mother who seemingly encouraged his father to take him to Freeman. Both step-mother and father accepted Freeman's advice that Dully needed surgery. Notwithstanding a series of previous medical opinions declaring Dully sane and some declaring the step-mother not sane, Freeman's judgement was that Dully was suffering from schizophrenia and had been seriously mentally disordered since early childhood.

So it was that a 12-year-old boy found himself being wheeled into an operating theatre to receive electric shocks as anaesthesia and have a metal device punched through his orbital cavities to cure him of his troubled and troubling mind. His step-mother and father received a bill of US$200 for the operation.

On awakening from the operation Dully recalls how he was feverish, had a severe headache, his eyes were swollen and bruised, and that he had no memory of what had happened to cause these physical effects. There were, however, to be more severe post-operative social sequelae for Dully. During the next four decades, Dully recollects that he was in the main either homeless or in mental hospitals, prisons or other types of institutions. During that time he became an alcoholic and drug-addicted. Freeman's ice-pick, certainly for the first 40 years, had not engineered much of a cure it would seem.

It was not, according to Dully, until 1998, at the age of 50, that his life changed for the better. By the time he co-authored his book, he described himself in terms of archetypal normality:

> My name is Howard Dully. I'm a bus driver. I'm a husband, and a father and a grandfather. I'm into doo-wop music, travel, and photography.
> *Dully and Fleming, 2008, p.ix*

He had sobered-up, married, procreated, gained an academic degree and succumbed to a heart attack, such was his normality.

Refined regulation

By the time Dully and Fleming published their book the conceptual and procedural crudity of mental medicine would appear to be waning, certainly if measured by the elaborate presentation of contemporary textbooks for psychiatrists (see as exemplar Hales *et al.*, 2014). Drugs and talking therapies have replaced spinning chairs and cold baths. Effective anaesthesia is used with electro-convulsive and surgical treatments, both of which have become tightly regulated. Old and new techniques became much more nuanced and mostly consented to, compared to Cotton and Freeman's versions although their use continues to be divisive even amongst psychiatrists (Kellner, 2011; Fisher, 2014).

The physical containment of patients by staff has moved from a frequent, rudimentary, and ferocious affair to a professed honed set of positive and skilled interventions set alongside strict health and safety guidelines and non-injurious equipment and settings to be instituted only *in extremis* (National Institute for Health and Care Excellence, 2015). Most, if not all psychiatric treatments are expected to adopt rigorous 'evidence-based' criteria acquired from rigorous empirical data ideally from randomised trials, laboratory experiments, or large-scale-representative surveys (WHO, 2013; Taylor, 2012).

Yet, the refinement of the means of reconfiguring the social script of people diagnosed with a mental disorder from that of abnormality to normality has not in essence altered their controlling properties (Morrall and Muir-Cochrane, 2002). Drugs are the mainstay of contemporary psychiatric treatment for those living in institutions or their own homes. If psychotherapy is offered and accepted then drugs may also be prescribed (Gabbard, 2009). A substantial aspect of psychotherapy and psycho-pharmaceuticals (as well as electro-convulsive-treatment) is adaptation. The general aim of both is to modify, with or without the conscious effort and accord of the recipient, or indeed the mindfulness of the donor, performance. The alteration of performance is mostly normative. It is adjusted towards a desirable state both for the individual but also society (Breggin, 2007; Morrall, 2008).

Moreover, the move away from Goffman's 'total institutions' with the advent of community care has not forestalled medical and legal intrusion into the lives of the mad. Mental health legislation in, for example, the USA, England and Australia, has at the same time as purporting to protect the human rights of the mad, reinforced the right of psychiatrists, and psychiatric nurses to supervise patients in the community, and enforce treatment possibly by enforced re-incarceration should either be deemed necessary by the professionals (Rosenberg, 2014; Hazelton and Morrall, 2016).

Rights and insights

Human liberty or rather the lack of it amongst nineteenth-century asylum patients, was a major motivating factor for Perceval to write about his experiences. He points out that being considered mad meant for him that liberties were taken with all aspects of his everyday life, including his freedom, and mostly without any rationale being offered:

> [M]en acted as though my body, soul, and spirit were fairly given up to their control, to work their mischief and folly upon.
> *Perceval in Bateson, 1962, p.112*

Perceval insightfully points out that his own use of violence ought not to mean that violence could be inflicted upon him. Perhaps the most incisive insight made by Perceval is the 'most blameable error' committed by the medical madhouse managers of placing mad people together in what might often be mayhem. It is, he reasons, wholly counterproductive to try to contain if not cure insanity by confining the insane in situations of insanity.

In May 1832 Perceval, somewhat less rebellious but still not a 'good patient' in the Goffman sense was removed from the Brislington Asylum and placed, once more against his will, in the asylum at Ticehurst in Sussex where he stayed until the beginning of 1834. As Porter notes, this second asylum, as with the first, was supposed to operate a compassionate ethos associated with the Quaker 'moral therapy'. However, according to Porter, Perceval's overall estimation of the second asylum was as nearly as negative as the first:

> Ticehurst House in Essex, possibly the most lavish private madhouse in the country, [was] run by Dr Charles Newington. Ticehurst proved scarcely better than Brislington. Here too he [Perceval] found himself being brutally manhandled by lower-class attendants he looked on as 'hinds' and 'clowns'.
>
> *Porter, 1987, pp.171–172*

Soon after his time spent in Brislington and Ticehurst, Perceval managed to be sane enough to get married and subsequently father four daughters, as well as write the two *Narrative* texts. Later he was to edit a book of poetry, and to champion the human rights of asylum inmates through his support for the 'Alleged Lunatics Friends Society', an advocacy group of and for the embryonic 'psychiatric survivors' movement (Bateson, 1962; Porter, 1987). He died in 1876 aged 73.

Gregory Bateson

The editor of *Perceval's Narrative*, Gregory Bateson (1904–1980), has similar views to those of Goffman about institutionalising the mad but these arise from his particular idea about the cause of madness rather than his view of asylums. Gregory Bateson's father was the eminent biologist William Bateson who furthered the work of Gregor Mendel (1822–1884) on genetic inheritance in humans. Mendel has come to be regarded as the founder of the science of genetics (Miko, 2008).

As far back as the early part of the nineteenth century, the medical specialist in mental maladies Esquirol (see Chapter 1) had suspicions that heredity played a part in the production of madness. Since then psychiatry has increasingly invested in attempting to clarify the specific genes which may predispose outbreaks of many serious mental disorders, and in particular schizophrenia (Trimble and George, 2010). All the more surprising that the son of a famous geneticist, and himself a biologist, should steer towards a psycho-social explanation of that particular madness. That is, he focuses on psychological and social factors rather than biological ones with regard to the causation of schizophrenia (Bateson *et al.*, 1956). Bateson's and his colleague's idea was to open-up opportunities for psychologists, sociologists, and renegade psychiatrists to conjecture on a multitude of similar factors which may be responsible for an underlying propulsion towards madness, rather than only substandard genes, bio-chemical discrepancies or anatomical brain defects.

Double-bind

The psycho-social idea on offer by Bateson with his collaborators (Bateson *et al.*, 1956) is based on data gained from studying the communication patterns of an unspecified number of patients diagnosed with schizophrenia, the written, verbal and taped accounts of psychotherapists and their own reflections when treating such patients, and from interviewing a small number of parents of schizophrenic patients. Bateson was well aware that their psycho-social idea was in need of much more rigorous empirical evidence than he had already obtained. His hypothesis he termed the 'double-bind'. A double-bind occurs during verbal and non-verbal interpersonal communication when one message is contradicted by another. The person receiving these messages is in a dilemma over how to respond because to reply to any is to be placed in the wrong. For Bateson, the psycho-social situation in which double-binds may trigger schizophrenia was the family, and the usual architect of the double-bind in the family was the mother.

Bateson suggested that whilst double-binds were common in human communications there were three key pathological characteristics in how the families of schizophrenics communicated. First, the mother may become anxious and hostile and subsequently withdraw her affections when her child seeks love from her. Second, this induces denial in the mother for what she unconsciously experiences as an unacceptable response, and implies blame on the child for not responding to her lovingly when she does ostensibly offer affection. Third, the father does not mediate between mother and child. For Bateson, this double-bind was much more common in the mother–male child relationship than in the mother–female child relationship. When this pathological communication becomes routine then schizophrenia may materialise in the child.

According to Bateson the reason that the affected child isn't able to communicate effectively and assertively to get out of the double-bind is twofold. First, it is very difficult for anyone to extract him/herself successfully from such communicative entanglements once they are deeply ingrained in the way the individuals concerned interact. Second, the family dynamics in which double-binds are perpetrated create an intense inter-dependency through which the child does not develop the acumen, skills or volition to overcome the predicament he/she is in.

What Bateson's double-bind hypothesis infers is that schizophrenia is a learned confusion in thinking and emotions rather than an inborn disorder which manifests as confused thoughts and emotions. The hypothesis was published in the 1950s and was radical then and remains so. It goes completely against the biological bents of contemporary psychiatry particularly in relation to schizophrenia. It is also radically 'politically incorrect' because it and ideas of a similar ilk (espoused for example by Ronald Laing – see Chapter 3) seem to lay the responsibility for this form of madness at the door of the family and especially pin-points mothers as causative. As Australian family psychotherapist Paul Gibney (2006, p.51) gently puts it '… that might offend today's sensibilities …'. But in defence of Bateson, he avers that to read Bateson's original idea as inferring families and mothers were wholly to blame for schizophrenia is 'the work of less skilled theorists' (Gibney, 2006, p.51).

Bateson sought in Percival's autobiographical recollections a theory to explain the cause of madness which differed from the dominant notions of psychiatry but nevertheless would be thought-out rigorously and underscored by empirical evidence. Moreover, he considers some of Perceval's thinking to be more than the subjective and embittered speculations of a madman, but semi-scientific and humane contributions understanding and managing madness. For example, Bateson recognises that Perceval discerned human consciousness as interconnected with an unconscious part of the mind, an understanding which pre-dated Freud's attempt to make this part of his scientific analysis of human psychology.

Listening and hearing

Bateson (1962) also appreciates and fostered Perceval's post-asylum campaigning for the voice of the mad person to be not only listened to but heard. Perceval's activism encompassed both the demand for the opinions of the mad to count if not dominate with regard to treatment and the conditions of care. He can, therefore, be considered as one of the first of those who were much later to describe themselves as 'psychiatric survivors', that is, patients who have, in their view, been mistreated within the psychiatric system (Morrison, 2013). Bateson's view on the mad talking back to psychiatry was to contribute considerably to the ideas of later 'anti-psychiatrists', although this was not always acknowledged (see Chapter 3).

However, far from Bateson endowing the voice of the mad person as the authority on his/her own madness as demanded by Perceval, he remained the expert in charge of explaining what it was the mad were actually saying and why they were saying what they said. Moreover, although Bateson 'listens' to the written words of Perceval, he used them not to promote the 'patient's point of view', a 'lay perspective', nor to help open-up some alternative theoretical consideration, but to shore-up his already established idea. Bateson's idea had been generated and circulated long before his analysis of Perceval was published. The internal melees expressed by Perceval provided evidential fodder for Bateson's pre-set explanation for the cause of schizophrenia. Bateson presides over Perceval's autobiographical descriptions and analyses, providing his judgements about what should be made of Perceval's words and thereby his mind.

Bateson was not the only reviewer of *Perceval's Narrative* who professed to want the mad to speak for themselves but who couldn't resist analysis. Porter, a promoter of stories of madness as told by the mad, offers a Freudian perspective replete with suspected Oedipal inferences:

> [P]erceval's own family background also seems particularly tailor-made for Freudian analysis: a father murdered while his son was but a child; a mother who quickly remarried, but who clearly remained the overwhelming focus for her unmarried son's love and loyalties ... The Oedipal ... echoes are strong.
>
> *Porter, 1987, p.173*

Perceval's view of his own mental state vacillated, sometimes considering himself assuredly mad, but at other times regarding the medical practitioners looking after him to be more insane than their patients, referring to them as the 'lunatic doctors' (Perceval in Bateson, 1962). Bateson's adjudication is that Perceval was most certainly mad much of the time if not perpetually and that doctors may be wrong-headed with regard to madness but they are not lunatics. Moreover, whilst claiming to be respectful of what it is the mad say about their lives and their mental conditions, Bateson not only supplants their opinions but with regard to Perceval's narration, he reveals a highly patronising attitude. He refers to the whole of the *Narrative* as 'the diatribes of a single patient' (Bateson, 1962, p.xii), and that Perceval must have been 'singularly uncomfortable to live with' (Bateson, 1962, p.xv). This is Bateson 'hearing' Perceval at a time when the latter considers himself not mad, that is years after his incarceration when he is writing the *Narrative*:

> How sane is the anger of a man [Perceval] who must repetitiously justify his anger? ... How sane is a man who must assert his intention to escape from a lunatic asylum before he makes the actual attempt?
>
> *Bateson 1962, p. 125*

Bateson then declares that the reasons for Perceval being difficult, ridden by anger and for his excessive rigidity and uprightness, were the very reasons for him eventually recovering. This interpretation is very odd. Bateson maintains that Perceval never recovered, or certainly not by the time he was writing the *Narrative* as is indicated in the above quotation.

Bateson's bind

There are many inconsistencies in Bateson's evaluation of Perceval's madness and by implication in his idea generally about madness. He commits himself to 'hearing' Perceval but then is disparaging overall about Perceval's account but admiring of parts. Furthermore, he doesn't explain why, when the crucial focus of his double-bind hypothesis is what happens in the family, little is made of the dynamics of Perceval's relationships with his siblings and parents. There are pathologies noted by Bateson in the family life of Perceval (particularly concerning the father's religiosity). However, these do not add up to Bateson's view on the cause of madness being specific and so psychologically toxic that they necessitate Perceval becoming what he describes as the 'necessary sacrifice' (Bateson, 1962, p.xviii). Perceval's mother seems to get off very lightly given mothers are usually for Bateson the catalyst for sending their sons insane.

Furthermore, Bateson adopts the medical label of schizophrenia but qualifies his acceptance of it as a real disorder in the medical sense without offering an alternative way of categorising the elements of human performance which becomes labelled in this way. Yet another inconsistency is in his claim that madness can be self-repairing. Why then bother to find causes or cures? Surely, Bateson should just have recommended 'time' for those who are not dangerous to themselves or others and for those who are, then 'time' in secure surroundings until they heal? That is, there is no need for therapeutic interference as suggested by Bateson (Bateson *et al.*, 1956) and advanced by a multitude of psycho-social devotees such as Gibney (2006).

But there is a further inconsistency with regard to interfering with a person's madness. Bateson states that madness 'must be regarded as disastrous', but then says that Perceval was: 'a better, happier, and more imaginative man after his psychotic experience' (Bateson, 1962, p.xx).

Is Bateson therefore caught in multiple-binds of his own making? Whether or not there are binds in Bateson's idea about insanity, some of Bateson's other empirical and intellectual work remains recognised, for example, through the awarding of an annual 'Gregory Bateson Prize' by the Society for Cultural Anthropology in the USA (SCA, 2015).

Andrew Scull

Andrew Scull (1947–) is a radical sociologist who has had what he describes as a 'life-long obsession' with the history of madness (2010). For over forty years he has researched the rise and fall of the asylums and the role of psychiatry in managing the mad. In doing so he has proffered the idea that power and social control are interlinked with the medicalisation of madness.

Much has already been mentioned already about power and control in this chapter and in Chapter 1. Andrew Scull (1977; 1979; 1993a; 1993b), however, takes a particular stance on control which relies heavily on the sociological implications from the work of Karl Marx. Marxist sociology proposes that society is structured in such a way as to benefit those who are in power or wish to gain power, installed or imminent ruling class (Feuer, 1978). Nationally and increasingly transnationally the powerful stratum maintains its power (its privileges, wealth and status) through the dual controlling mechanisms of ideology and coercion. That is, the inculcation of the population with the belief that the powerful deserve their power combined with the threat or actual exercising of force keeps power in the grip of the already powerful or enables the aspirational (Giddens and Sutton, 2013; Le Blanc, 2016).

When this structuralist approach from sociology is applied by Scull to psychiatry then it is viewed as colluding with the ruling class. The former performs as an 'agency of social control' on behalf of the latter. The police, the judiciary, the army, the clergy and school teachers, function very obviously to regulate – or at least attempt so to do – individuals and society overall. Psychiatrists take charge of madness on behalf of the ruling stratum because the thoughts, behaviours and emotions of the mad are considered to deviate from what the rulers want to perpetuate, for their own advantage, as acceptable performance.

Capitalism and asylumdom

Hence, from Scull's perspective, psychiatry is not freeing the mad from their disorders but subjugating a seditious segment of society. By extension, this Marxist approach implies that within the globalising capitalist system of economic production of the twenty-first century the potency of corporate executives, politicians, bankers and the wealthy, continues to be aided by controlling activities of psychiatry.

Scull (1979) regards the large-scale building of special institutions in which to house the mad as a momentous means of controlling the mad, which accords with the view of the non-Marxist Foucault (see Chapter 1). The powerful through mass incarceration sought to remove this element of the socially deviant from the general population. That the mad in these institutions were to become managed by the medical profession was down to its good fortune and clever occupational tactics which resulted in the birth of a sub-speciality focusing on the mental rather than the physical. The consequence of this take-over of the asylums by the medical profession was the medicalisation of madness. Scull (as does Foucault) recognises that this movement to control madness by the powerful (which he names 'asylumdom') was part of an overall move to increase the institutional containment of other social deviants amongst whom were the workless and work-shy, the impoverished, epileptics, idiots and imbeciles (previous legal terms for people with learning disabilities), as well as criminals.

Where Scull and Foucault differ is over timing and justification. For Foucault, certainly in France, the 'Great Confinement' of the mad happened during the seventeenth and eighteenth centuries. For Scull the nineteenth century was the real 'Age of Confinement':

> All across Western Europe and North America, a veritable mania for the construction of the new institutions for the insane marked the middle decades of the 19th century.
>
> *Scull, 2011, p.49*

Foucault places an emphasis on the moral threat of the mad to the scruples of the emerging bourgeoisie which triggered the policy of incarceration. In particular, the work ethic was undermined by the mad and hence was to provide the rationale for treatment to be based on training the inmates of institutions to be diligent. Scull refers to the perceived economic threat of madness to the rapidly industrialising and urbanising economies of Europe. The new economic mode needed a major renovation of working practices from those associated with agriculture. These included highly regimented work in terms of the length, pattern and intensity of the working day, a change to the location of work from the land to the factory, and living arrangements shifting from rudimentary rural housing to unsanitary, disease-ridden and over-crowded town slums.

Friedrich Engels was the friend, the benefactor of and collaborator with, Marx in his quest to demystify the realities of the capitalist economic system (Hunt, 2010). Engels published his personal account of the reality of the conditions in which the working class (and those not able to find work) was living when the industrial revolution, the engine of the capitalist economic system, was fully underway in the 1840s. He provides stark description of observations from his wanderings around England's 'great towns':

> [T]he stronger treads the weaker underfoot, and the powerful few, the capitalists, seize everything for themselves, while the weak many, the poor, scarcely a bare existence remains … [M]any have died of starvation, where long continued want of proper nourishment has called forth fatal illness.
>
> *Engels, 1969, original 1845, pp.58–59*

Fear about the mad and madness by early in the nineteenth century, argues Porter (1987), had been stoked to the point that it verged on hysteria. The political authorities, entrepreneurs, industrialists and nascent practitioners of mental medicine, warned the public that the emerging industrial fabric (economic and/or moral) could be damaged by those who could not or would not fit into its associated imposts. They gave notice that a return to savagery could be the outcome if social deviants such as the mad were not removed from the normal population.

Opportunities and privileges

So the medical profession for Scull was an active and eager partner in a plot devised by those in power to control the mad. The particularly powerful in the industrial era were the capitalists, the owners of the means of industrial production. Psychiatry assisted in building-up and maintaining the capitalist structure of society because this serves them well in terms of their occupational goals of elevated social ranking and associated augmented remuneration.

However, for Foucault (1966) and another notable non-Marxist social thinker, Max Weber (1978; original 1922), who is one of the founders of sociology as an academic subject (Radkau, 2011), power in society is diversified. That is, power is not (only) in the hands of one unified elite section. Groups from throughout society compete with each other to gain prestige and prosperity. Psychiatry and the medical profession generally have done rather well through its leading proponents shrewd occupational strategies. These have, over centuries allowed its membership to, in Foucault's terms (2006), 'enjoy' power for its patent and direct rewards rather than, in Scull's terms, primarily acting as a conduit to supply power to the (capitalist) ruling class.

An aim of the World Psychiatric Association, which represents 200,000 psychiatrists from 117 countries, is:

> To be a voice for the dignity and human rights of the patients and their families, *and to uphold the rights of psychiatrists.* [emphasis added]
>
> *WPA, 2016*

This espoused ambition of the World Psychiatric Association (WPA) implies that psychiatrists are entitled to their trade and justified to trade their interpretations of madness.

The WPS offers alternative conceptualisations of madness to that of standard Western-leaning psychiatry. For example, it has a 'Transcultural Section' within which culturally-sensitive adjustments are considered, and whether or not the latest latest Diagnostic and Statistical Manual of Mental Disorders (DSM) has spawned inappropriate categories and the over-medicalisation of madness has been debated in its journal *World Psychiatry* (Frances, 2013a). Furthermore, an editorial about the political mission of the profession has been published in which action is called for to deal with social factors affecting mental health:

> What contributes to poor mental health is well known (1): adverse childhood conditions; experience of war, persecution and torture (2); social isolation; unemployment and social exclusion; poverty, poor education and low socio-economic status; and social inequality.
>
> *Priebe, 2015*

Self-criticism and unconventional polemics, however, are not only sporadic in such journals but arguably are tokenistic because their effect in undermining the main medicalised thrust of psychiatric expansionism would appear to be negligible. As with the 'moral' approach during the age of asylumdom, alternative therapies can be integrated into the dominant perspective. In the main, this dominant perspective is reinforced by the journal of the WPA. The journal concentrates on psychiatric orthodoxy and applying that orthodoxy across social groups and globally through 'hard' scientific research. For example, in the same issue of the WPS journal as the above call for the politicisation of psychiatry, articles appear with the following titles:

- Cardiovascular and cerebrovascular risk factors and events associated with second-generation antipsychotic compared to antidepressant use – results from a claims-based inception cohort study;
- Prevalence of psychiatric disorders in U.S. older adults: findings from a nationally representative survey in a non-elderly adult sample;
- Cyberchondria, cyberbullying, cybersuicide, cybersex: 'new' psycho-pathologies for the 21st century?

In a 2013 educational video link on the website of the British Royal College of Psychiatrists to what is presented as the historical timeline of psychiatry, there is no mention of anything other than the relentlessly enlightened, humane and scientific innovativeness of medical practice in the field of madness. The narrator refers to the long history of medical involvement in madness stretching from the work of Islamic physicians in the eighth century through to the 'promising' work of twenty-first century Western-orientated and heavily technical and biologically-based psychiatrists. The fruits of neuropsychology, neuroimaging, neurochemistry, psycho-pharmacology and genetics, are acclaimed, as is psychiatry as a speciality for medical students (its target audience) on qualifying:

> So with all the recent advances the future [of psychiatry, its scientific insights, technologies and treatments] is looking very promising, *and there are lots of opportunities for people moving into this field* to really make fundamental discoveries about the nature of psychiatric illnesses. [emphasis added]
>
> *Royal College of Psychiatrists, 2013*

Moreover, the narrator in the above video calls the discovery of the first wave of anti-psychotic drugs during the mid-twentieth century the 'big break' in the effectiveness of physical methods of treatment (electro-convulsive-therapy is also regarded in a positive light), and unequivocally connects this with the emptying of the mental hospitals.

Places of refuge

Asylumdom, Scull argues, materialised for economic reasons (that is, capitalism and the capitalists required it to be done) not as a consequence of medical philanthropy or their therapeutic accomplishment. Scull (1997) also argues that care in the community re-materialised for an economic reason. The prevention of admission to and emptying of the mental hospitals, what Scull calls 'decarceration', began to happen in earnest from the 1950s onwards in England and in most other industrialised countries around this time (Busfield, 1986; 2011). However, Scull (1977) argues that just as incarceration did not happen because of the onward progression of psychiatry, neither did decarceration.

Medical historian Edward Shorter (1997) espouses the version of the history of doctors' engagement with madness as steadily more scientific, more humane and more successful. He traces the progression of psychiatry from before the asylums to the point at which the second wave of major anti-psychotic drugs and the happiness-inducing pill, Prozac, became available. Shorter gives support to the idea that the asylums were for many mad people better than living with their families or wandering alone from village to village.

According to Shorter's account of the history of psychiatry, people received into the asylums were found regularly to be in a terrible state following years of ill-treatment at the hands of their relatives. One youth from Bavaria had been kept in a pig pen by his father. He ate from a bowl by lapping-up the food as would an animal. Another, in Ireland, was kept for years until his death in a low-level pen hollowed-out in the floor of a peasant's cottage. The top of the pen was covered with a grill to prevent escape and through which he would have been fed. Tethering was an alternative to caging:

> One [German] man had been chained by his wife to the wall of their house for five years, losing the use of his legs … In England, such patients, if not chained at home, might be fastened to a stake in a workhouse or poorhouse.
>
> *Shorter, 1997, p.3*

Shorter comments that many of those admitted into the asylums would have signs of having been beaten routinely. Asylums were, for Shorter, to offer the mad what the word literally means, a place of refuge.

But, the reputation of these refuges has come to be one of condemnation, not approbation. That the mad in the nineteenth century usually went to their refuge by force or the threat of force and without any choice over where was to be their haven, and that this haven turned out to be somewhat less than a salutary experience, continues to be the common view (see, for example: Rutherford 2008; Davis, 2013; Wise, 2013). Dully's experiences of various 'mental' institutions in the subsequent century, let alone his encounter with the pick-axe wielding Freeman, can't easily be regarded as conferring refuge.

One sort of institution or another in which the mad were incarcerated (for example, in gaols, guard-houses, or workhouses) had existed for centuries. The religious order of St. Mary of Bethlehem in London used its priory built in 1247, initially to house the homeless, then people with intellectual restrictions or epilepsy. About a century later it started to accept the mad (Andrews *et al.*, 1997). Bethlem has stood out in the social history of madness as representing all that was wrong with institutional care for the mad. Its ignominious character in the public imagination persisted from when it started to accept the mad, continuing over hundreds of years to represent harsh living conditions, cruel treatment and the hopelessness of mental derangement once it takes hold. On the finding of thousands of skeletons of Bethlem's inmates buried in a 500-year-old graveyard, dug-up to make way for a new railway, a tabloid newspaper journalist exemplifies popular opinion:

> They were the tortured souls incarcerated in the world's first mental asylum. The uproar, chaos and barbarism that surrounded them gave the place its famous nickname, which has resonated for centuries as a byword for madness – Bedlam.
>
> *MaCrae, 2013*

But is this a fair declamation of all of Bethlem and asylumdom overall? Historian Catherine Arnold (2008) argues that it is not.

The exact date when the mad were first admitted to Bethlem is uncertain, although it is generally accepted as being during the fourteenth century (Andrews *et al.*, 1997). Arnold suggests it was in the 1370s when it would be little better than a ramshackle hovel built over an area in which human excrement flowed out of blocked sewage pipes. However, agreeing with Shorter's position about what incarceration offered the mad Arnold posits that at least Bethlem gave a modicum of shelter and safety for those people who had not the mental capacity or material resources to cope with what she submits was a hostile outside world.

Unlike later asylums where once admitted inmates may indeed have spent the rest of their lives, Bethlem had for most of its mad population a 'one-year-rule'. This suggests an unprecedented fast and effective mending of madness at Bethlem. However, the intention behind the one-year-rule' was to avoid Bethlem becoming a place for chronic cases. Buildings were erected at Bethlem for 'incurables', but most inmates, whether still mad or not, were discharged back into the hostile world from whence they came (Andrews *et al.*, 1997).

Museums of madness

Other western European countries had designated a few institutions for the mad by the beginning of the Renaissance. In regions of the Rhine, which would later become part of Germany, and the states which these groups were also collected and put in a variety of old buildings (Porter, 1987). A similar pattern of sporadic internment occurred in the hotchpotch of polities which eventually were to be incorporated into what was to become Italy (Scull, 2015).

In France, from the middle of the seventeenth century, Scull (2015) notes, the nobility in France had become worried that a growth in the population of the poor, the idle and vagrants might threaten their hold on power. The main place of incarceration in Paris was the Hôpitaux Généraux where amongst disparate inmates were some of the mad. However, Scull's position is that the use of institutions to house the mad was irregular, and usually the choice of last resort rather than representing of mass sequestration of the insane (2015). Crucially, for Scull's thesis about the mass incarceration of the mad having been driven by major economic changes related to industrialisation is that in France, Germany, Italy, and especially in England only a small proportion of the mad even by the end of the eighteenth century were placed in such institutions. Moreover, in England at that time they were attended by only a few dozen medical practitioners. The few specialist institutions for the mad which did exist (for example the French *petite maisons* and English madhouses) admitted only tens of patients. According to Scull, no matter the magnitude of its reputation as a place of Bedlam, Bethlem's mad population size was only around 50 for much of its early history (Scull, 1993a).

Mass sequestration of the mad began in earnest in England with the passing of the 1845 Lunacy Act. This legislation forced local authorities to provide special institutions for the mad. There followed the massive public building programme of asylums. The in-patient numbers in Britain rose from approximately 5,000 at the beginning of the nineteenth century to 100,000 at the beginning of the twentieth century. As the era of mass institutional care was coming to an end in the 1950s, the asylums, by then renamed mental hospitals, had an overall inmate population of about 150,000 (Porter, 1987). These 'museums of madness' to use another of Scull's inimitable phrases, had become small towns, with a social structure and economy all of their own, and in which not only thousands of patients lived but so did hundreds of staff. Many employees resided within the grounds of these institutions and spent much of their leisure time there. The asylums and then the mental hospitals had indeed become Goffman's total institutions.

For the writers of the orthodox history of psychiatry such as Shorter (1997), whilst the asylums had been the progressive alternative to an absence of, or to meagre or brutish provision, the next progressive stage in managing the mad was for the mad to go back to, or to remain in, the community. That is, the asylum epoch had been functional for about 150 years but its course had been run and another epoch of care was to take over as the next step in the enduring progress of psychiatry. It is worth reflecting, however, that the majority of countries in the world throughout the nineteenth and twentieth centuries had never shifted from community care, albeit mainly rudimentary and not necessarily very caring (Morrall and Hazelton, 2004).

Psycho-pharmacology

The foremost factor instigating the policy of closing the large mental hospitals continues to be cited as the result of advancements made, mostly surreptitiously, in pharmacology (Marston, 2013). Chief amongst the mind-altering drugs being manufactured to re-energise psychiatry was the discovery of the anti-psychotic Largactil (Chlorpromazine). This major tranquilliser did just that. It allowed patients diagnosed with schizophrenia to be tranquil enough to be discharged and stopped those who hadn't yet entered the mental hospital from so doing or if they did become an in-patient then this was only for a short period.

According to Scull (2015), however, it is not the mad who have benefitted from drugs but psychiatry. Psychiatry's power and expansion, he argues, has been aided and abetted by the pharmaceutical industry. The drug companies have supplied huge amounts of money for research and spent massive sums on marketing their products when the outcomes of the research indicate that these are effective. Medical conferences are festooned with literature and replete with gifts aimed at encouraging their attendees to prescribe particular medication. Some medical journals are underwritten by the companies, and most medical journals carry stylish adverts to inform and then entice practitioners to prescribe their products. The pharmaceutical industry is also accused by Scull of providing validation, if only implicitly and obliquely, for the 2013 version of the DSM, and, for him, its near catch-all sweep of all of human performance.

Underscoring his attack on psychiatry and the immodest account of its history and efficacy, Scull (2015) refers to the heavy toll paid through the serious side-effects of the drugs on offer to the mad. He also points to what he considers to be the astonishing realisation that the life expectancy of those with serious mental disorder has declined in recent times. This for Scull is because of the negative effect the later range of drugs has on metabolism which results in higher than average rates of diabetes, weight gain and heart disease. The older drugs were replaced because of other undesirable impacts on health including blurred vision, fast heart rate, low blood pressure, urinary retention, constipation and uncontrollable movements of the muscles.

Medication throughout medical practice has also come under intense scrutiny by medical practitioner Ben Goldacre (2012). Goldacre has accused what he refers to as 'Bad Pharma' of misleading patients and the public about the therapeutic worth of a wide range of their products. He argues that his medical colleagues, including psychiatrists, are at best also duped by, or at worse collude in, what for him amounts to deceit. In accord with Scull, Goldacre argues that global pharmaceutical companies massage the way research into their products is conducted and disseminated, and use all sorts of tangible enticements and marketing gimmickry to seduce prescribers into picking their pills instead of their competitors or alternative (non-drug) treatments.

Perversely, it may be that the drug industry's interest in drugging the mad is faltering. It has been noted by Christian Fibiger (2012), who has held many senior scientific posts in the pharmaceutical industry, that psycho-pharmaceutical innovation has not been apparent since the latter part of the twentieth century. He explains that most of the large pharmaceutical companies have either decreased or abandoned their research and development into finding novel psychiatric drugs to concentrate on more profitable ventures such as cancer treatments. Fibiger recommends a resurgence of investment by the companies to instigate what he refers to as an 'exciting march' towards the invention of new drugs rather than an alternative non-pharmaceutical approach.

Economic determinism

According to Scull (1977) the march of psychiatry with its chemical remedies was not what revived care in the community. His economic deterministic argument is consistent when applied to the ending of asylumdom. Just as the economy (that is, the fast pace of industrialisation, urbanisation, and the formation of the capitalist mode of production) had been the catalyst for depositing a range of deviants into social silos, the shift from institutional care back to community care was propelled by economics.

What Scull contends is that a fiscal crisis occurring at the time resulted in the warehousing of the mad becoming too expensive to maintain. Most had been built a hundred years previously and the upkeep of the grounds and multiple buildings, some of which were deliberately – and expensively – constructed to be impressive and imposing architectural manifestations of the power of the State and psychiatry was beginning to be untenable for cash-strapped governments. There was an inexorable increase in the budget for staff as the professional status of doctors grew and nurses fought for comparable occupational headway, as well as higher staff numbers from a variety of non-medical/nursing disciplines. The latter included occupational therapists, clinical psychologists and social workers. This meant that each year increasingly more money was necessary to fund this way of handling insanity. Decamping the mad into the community, or rather not allowing them to be housed in the first place (which was what essentially had brought down the numbers in the mental hospitals significantly), was therefore considered a financially viable option. Cheaper accommodation would be made available in the community in the form of, for example, hostels and group-homes. An even cheaper option would be for families to continue with, or take-over, caring for their mad relatives.

But, not much of the money saved from the closing and selling-off of the mental hospitals found its way into the coffers of the local authorities who were responsible for the costs of caring in the community. The lack of resources made available to the community meant that many of the mad in North America, western Europe, and Australia, ended up in low-grade bed-and-breakfast accommodation, criminalised, unemployed, homeless, socially isolated, and their disorder and treatment left unsupervised (Brown, 1985; Bean and Mounser, 1993; Leff, 2001).

To his credit, Scull (1977) had warned of this side-effect of decarceration. That said, community care officially remains the main way to manage madness. The marginalisation and impoverishment of the mad after decarceration predicted by Scull has come to include the under-resourcing of both the remaining in-patient facilities and community services in the UK and USA (Gilburt, 2015; Honberg *et al.*, 2011).

Philanthropy and humanitarianism

The problem with both Shorter's and Scull's analysis is that they are too tapered to their respective primary perspective with regard to why institutional care and community care happened and to the disposition of psychiatry. A more rounded idea comes from sociologists Peter Miller and Nikolas Rose (1986). They accept that the State did set the tone for segregating the mad (for example in England through the 1845 Lunacy Act), but it had been propagated by private entrepreneurs much earlier. But, they argue, the planning of and paying for, mass incarceration was not, at least in the beginning, centralised but organised locally.

Moreover, they dispute Scull's and Foucault's notion that the mad were excluded from society fundamentally because they were considered by those in power to be a bad example to the overall population. From the point of view of the powerful, so Scull and Foucault suggest, the mad were social deviants either because they threatened the moral order (Foucault) or the capitalist mode of production (Scull). But Miller and Rose point to philanthropic and humanitarian ideals which led to the building of many of the asylums in England, France, Germany and the USA. Local dignitaries and medical practitioners wanted to protect the mad from what could be appalling living conditions in the community.

Shorter (1997) implies that given the conditions in which the mad would otherwise have had to live with their families or roam the land, being inside an asylum with medical overseers may not have been such an appalling option. Having a roof over their heads with food supplied, gave some compensation for enduring physical restraint, cold baths, hot baths, rotating mechanisms, bloodletting, purges and emetics. Whilst Miller and Rose are not agreeing with Shorter's enthusiastic take on the benefits of the medical profession medicalising madness they accept that asylumdom and the emergence of psychiatry in the asylums bestowed better conditions on many of the mad than they would otherwise have experienced. That the asylums also institutionalised, and instigated oppression, cruelty and crude social control, was an accidental outcome of benevolence not the planned product of malevolence, an example of the law of unintended consequences.

Miller and Rose along with Porter, also point out that the asylums in England had not been built either by or for the medical profession. This was not the case in France where Esquirol had championed institutional care (see Chapter 1). But in England, doctors were invited by local municipal leaders to oversee the administration of the new mad houses. Furthermore, occupational advancement for the medical profession may have become predicated on taking the opportunity afforded by the large-scale exclusion of the mad, but not to the exclusion of sincere attempts to soothe their suffering.

Alternative therapies

Alternative types of institutions to what Scull describes as 'warehouses' were built in France, the USA, Italy and England. Lay benefactors and religious groups such as the Quakers wanted 'moral therapy' to replace the medically dominated asylums and physical methods of treatment as well as the implied cruelty (Bynum et al., 1988). Moral management of the mad posited that an individual could be brought back to reason if handled more humanely:

[The moral therapy] movement aimed in effect to revive the dormant humanity of the mad, by treating them as endowed with a residuum at least of normal emotions, still capable of excitation and training ... They needed to be treated essentially like children, who required a stiff dose of rigorous discipline, rectification and retraining.

Porter, 1987, p.19

Training for work was considered pivotal to the mission of the moral therapists. Work was in itself regarded as moral. Tautologically, the movement's advocates argued this was because idleness was suspected of leading to immorality. Ways of indoctrinating the otherwise work-shy or work-incapable with the work ethic defined the daily life of the patient. Was this therefore any better in terms of control than medicalising the mad? The mad were not being dipped, spun, electrocuted, or drugged but their performance was still being regulated.

The asylums in which Perceval was placed were supposed to be ideal in extolling the ideals of moral therapy. His experience of moral therapy, however, appears to have been at variance with those ideals. He was taken for walks but doesn't mention being invited to work. Nor does he mention many examples of kindliness by those he considers to be not his therapists but his captors.

When alternatives to standard medical positions arise then the profession acts to defend its kudos and practice provinces, be they surgical, pharmaceutical, callisthenic, aromatic or psychological. If not antagonism (in particular condemning the would-be alternative for the lack of scientific evidential underpinning), then the occupational technique of absorption may be implemented (Morrall, 2009).

After much (mutual) antagonism, moral treatment was integrated within the medically run nineteenth century asylums alongside physical methods (Bynum *et al.*, 1988). Eventually, the medical managers of the asylums, and then the mental hospitals, would prescribe 'work' (which in the twentieth century morphed into 'occupational therapy' and 'industrial therapy') alongside cold baths, spinning chairs, seclusion and restraint.

Assimilation continued with the embracement first of Freudian thoughts and practices (see Chapter 1), and later those of social therapists. Social therapy, whereby the importance of interpersonal relationships, family and community, to the maintenance of mental health is recognised, have been a legitimised if peripheral form of psychiatric practice in the field since the mid-twentieth century (Clark, 1975). The 'therapeutic community' as a treatment for mental disorder, based on an equalisation of power between professionals and patients in a residential setting, was fostered in Britain by psychiatrist, Maxwell Jones (1953). Latterly, cognitive-behavioural therapy has been embraced as a legitimate psychiatric treatment for, i.e., personality disorder (Sperry and Sperry, 2015).

Female maladies

Many of these psychological and sociological ideas observe Miller and Rose (1986) came to the forefront around the same time as community care as a policy for the mad was coming to prominence offering an alternative to the large mental hospital. They also fitted a post-Second World War public demand for social change and the subsequent liberalisation with regard to attitudes towards human rights generally and in particular access to further and higher education, alternative lifestyles, drug-taking, sexuality and the role of women.

Regarding the latter, Denise Russell (1995), who adopts a feminist approach which has undertones of sociological structuralism, points out that by the end of the nineteenth century both public and private asylums contained more women than men. She argues that what she refers to as 'biological psychiatry' has done more harm than good and therefore it has harmed women more than men. Women who were poor and unmarried mothers were admitted to the asylums because the social circumstances of impoverishment or giving birth out of wedlock was considered depraved no matter what the woman's actual state of derangement.

This disparity continued into the twentieth century. Barbara Taylor (2014), Professor of Humanities at London University and feminist activist, was admitted into a large London mental hospital before all were closed in England during the 1990s. Where Taylor was admitted to Friern mental hospital, the ratio she calculates was 1.41 women for every 1 man. Moreover, she suggests that women were handled in the asylums differently to men. Perceived by staff to be more disruptive and malicious than men they were five times more likely to be given sedation, cold baths and placed in padded cells than male patients.

Both Russell and Taylor argue that psychiatry operating in the asylums and mental hospitals regarded women as having an inherent biological deficiency. That is, women, particularly those in the middle-class and upper-class tiers of western European and North American societies, were considered to be liable to madness merely because they were women. Their sexuality was especially suspected of being bothersome to their minds. However, Robert Burton, social commentator and cleric, writing in the seventeenth century had theorised that 'noble virgins', 'nice gentlewomen', widows and nuns, were in part prone to melancholy (depression) due to a stifling of their natural passions. He suggests a cure for these frustrated females:

> [T]he best and surest remedy of all, is to see them well placed, and married, to good husbands.
>
> *Burton, 2004, original 1624, p.100*

But there is for Russell and Taylor a need to look beyond the individual to understand psychological distress. Scull's (2012) 'disturbing history' of hysteria points to the interplay of social contexts, attitudes to gender and madness. As

Scull discusses, Freud's derogatory conceptualisation of women as biologically-driven psycho-social imperfection compared to men cannot be separated from Victorian perceptions of gender. Moreover, the apparent misogyny of Freud and that of his mentor the neurologist Jean-Martin Charcot is disputable given that both expressed views and engaged in professional practice which gave sustenance to loosening the societal shackles which controlled women's sexuality and their intellectual, and vocational progress (Young-Bruehl, 1990; Goetz, 1999).

For Russell and Taylor, together with other writers adopting a structural-feminist approach to 'female maladies' (for example, Showalter, 1987), the diagnosing of hysteria as well as depression much more amongst women than men during the nineteenth and twentieth centuries can be attributed specifically to the patriarchal structure of society and its attendant oppression of women by male-led psychiatry. By extension this argument could explain why in the twenty-first century depression along with other diagnostic categories such as anxiety, which have become by far the most common of mental disorders, continue to apply to women more than men (WHO, 2015). Conversely, given that the global rate of diagnosis of all mental disorder for men and women is nearly equal (*ibid*) it may be that oppression is a common feature or an irrelevant one.

For sociologist Joan Busfield (1996), Professor of Sociology at the University of Essex, UK, the relevant feature is power. The unequal structure of power between men and women in society as a whole which leads to negative or positive perceptions is replicated within the arenas in which madness is managed. However, as Busfield observes, power disparities also occur within genders. Such disparity in the nineteenth century resulted in Perceval's admission to more prestigious asylums than would have happened had his family been poor and powerless.

Fiscal flaw

For Miller and Rose (1986) mid-twentieth-century psychiatry was liberalising within the context of wider changes in how society was operating rather than independently moving along progressively as Shorter (1997) would have it. The availability of new anti-psychotic medication for schizophrenia, manic-depression and depression eased the passage of community care rather than creating it.

Asylumdom required considerable financial investment by local authorities and the State. As noted above, this investment was not replicated to ensure that community care worked effectively. Miller and Rose accept that there was in the UK fiscal concern about how the asylums could continue to exist given that they had grown enormously and the cost of maintaining them had escalated.

However, Miller and Rose spot a crucial flaw in Scull's economic deterministic argument for the demise of asylumdom and the rise of community care. They point out that the financial crisis did not occur certainly in the UK until decades after community care was under way. Scull, therefore, places far too much emphasis on decarceration having arisen as a consequence of national economic strife. Undoubtedly, the large mental hospitals were expensive to run but this was not the only or the overriding reason for their closure.

What Miller and Rose also point out is that the demise of the large mental hospital was fostered by a wave of reports and inquiries by journalists and social scientists about cruelty and neglect by mental hospital staff. Conversely, for Taylor (2014) the asylums were indubitably a place of refuge for those (men and women) suffering from severe mental distress. Notwithstanding the excesses taking place within them, Taylor mourns their passing as this function has not been replaced in the community.

Perceval's family was sufficiently well-off to have him taken care of within their midst. His relatives having decided this was not what they wanted for him or themselves at least ensured that his conditions – albeit with beatings and fetters – was better than most of those who were left to their own or their families' devices and to those who were incarcerated.

Unfettered control

No matter where the mad were, however, for Scull they faced from the nineteenth century onwards cumulating regulation. But, there is nothing inherently wrong morally or politically with social control unless adopting an extreme libertarian perspective (see Chapter 3). The most extreme libertarian believes in the freedom of the individual from most forms of control by the State or its agencies. It may, however, be difficult to conjure a society in which unfettered self-interest with little or no communal identity and responsibility is the norm.

The 'compact' balancing of individual freedom and social control was acclaimed and pondered in the days of the sophists in ancient Greece and most conspicuously by the eighteenth-century philosopher Jean-Jacques Rousseau (Cole, 1973). It continues to be discussed by governments and influences government policies in many countries (see for example, *The Economist*, 2015; Department of Health, 2015).

Most functioning societies can only function because they control individual freedom to a greater or lesser extent. Fascist and communist governments in practice attempt to control their populations to a great extent whilst liberal democracies in principle do so to a lesser extent. There is, therefore, an implicit or explicit social contract which operates to mediate between the needs and wants of the individual and those of the collective. Where control by the State has collapsed or been undermined severely then not only disorder but death and destruction can be the consequence. Latterly, dozens of countries have been listed by the nonpartisan research and educational organisation Fund for Peace (2015) as 'fragile'. South Sudan, Sudan, Somalia and the Central African Republic are regarded as the most fragile. Should fragility turn into fracture and failure then there is no society as happened with Yugoslavia. Where there is unfettered control by the State and its agencies, as in North Korea under the familial line of Comrade Kim Il Sung and Cambodia under the Khmer Rouge, then there can be equally disastrous results such as indoctrination and genocide (Morrall, 2006).

Unfettered control in psychiatry brought with it a disastrous consequence in the shape of forced sterilisation. Now considered a crime against humanity by the International Criminal Court (2016), this form of eugenics was legalised by the United States Supreme Court in the 1920s in certain circumstances, and carried out in many states in the USA by doctors working in prisons and mental hospitals until the 1970s (Black, 2012; Stern, 2005). The most obvious and odious example of eugenics on a genocidal scale is the Nazi German government's extermination of, amongst others, Jews, Gypsies and psychiatric patients. The latter, in a bizarre coming together of caring and killing, was with the cooperation of psychiatrists and psychiatric nurses (Foth, 2013).

The Nazis and what Scull (2015) regards as their enthusiastic supporters from within German psychiatry committed themselves to exterminating the mad. During the 1930s the Nazi Party had recruited approximately 50 per cent of all German medical practitioners, with psychiatrists over-represented compared with other specialities. Over 70,000 mentally disordered patients in the two years following the outbreak of the Second World War were killed using lethal injections and then the gas chambers. Around a quarter of a million mentally disordered patients were to be killed before the end of the war with only a very small number of German psychiatrists objecting to this genocide.

The 'scientific rationale' for the holocaust against the Jews was extracted from the lessons learned from the mass murder of the mad (Read and Dillon, 2013). Some of the psychiatrists and psychiatric nurses who were experienced in killing their patients were to participate in the holocaust (Read and Dillon, 2013). Moreover, psychiatry has been directly involved in political control in some countries, For example, the Soviet Union and Chinese ruling parties used the institutional provisions of psychiatry as unintended *de facto* prisons for dissidents (Bonnie, 2002).

Summary

Perceval's Narrative is a rich and candid description of madness, and provides one inmate's personal experience at the birth of the asylum as the main way of managing the mad and the birthing of psychiatry as a suitable sphere for medical participation and subsequently the wholesale medicalisation of madness.

Perceval was placed in small privately run and relatively affluent asylums. As Porter (1987) observes, for those placed in the early public madhouses prior to the asylum movement and for many years after it had got underway, beatings and binding were not unusual but commonplace. The inmates, suggests Porter, may not have been treated any better in the latter than they would have been if they had been animals. However, some of the mad were treated no better than animals (assuming that in those days animals were treated badly) when they were living outside of the asylums. Left to wander the fields and hedgerows or shackled in a barn or cellar, their lives resembled that of entrapped beasts. The building of the asylums had not been at the behest of the profession of medicine but had allowed the profession to extend its interest in maladies of the mind and to build up its physical methods of treatment as well as its occupational dominance. Thereby the sub-discipline of psychiatry was crafted.

Goffman points out that these 'total institutions' and their medical managers also crafted the mad into the role of the 'good patient' who had to conform to being mad and then to being sane. Only if the mad played-out this institutional script could they hope to be discharged. Bateson applies his 'double-bind' hypothesis to examine what might bring the mad to the attention of those wishing to initiate incarceration, specifically the initial cause of the medicalised category of schizophrenia. He argues that this form of madness is a sane reaction to insane communicative processes within the family (and more of this hypothesis in Chapter 3). Scull provides a Marxist critique of psychiatry aimed at unmasking its function as an agency of social control on behalf of the ruling class, and this approach has been revived by other sociologists (for example: Cohen, 2016).

Perceval's Narrative is obviously subjective and written by him years after the events he describes occurred. There are no accounts written by his family, his doctors or by other inmates to serve as comparators to Perceval's *Narrative*. Moreover, if Perceval was indeed mad then his madness forms another – for better or worse in terms of precision – interpretative prism.

Recalling what is and isn't accurate about events which occurred much earlier is problematic for everyone. Memory is fallible and fabrication inevitable (Kahneman, 2011). Dully has provided invaluable autobiographical commentary about being a child-patient of a psychiatrist experimenting with surgical treatments during the mid-twentieth century. He, however, has the added disadvantage with regard to recall of having had an 'ice-pick' lobotomy. Dully admits that his memory is hazy, not helped by the competing narratives he has collected relating to his psychiatric experiences (Dully quoted in Grimes, 2007).

Perceval, despite being placed amongst the insane had become psychologically sound and had eventually become an archetypal 'good patient' and 'good citizen'. Dully, despite or perhaps because of being surgically brutalised has become mentally healthy and socially respectable. Both, however, were to use their sanity to protest lucidly about the types of institutions and interventions, which it could be claimed, had helped to make their sanity and lucid protestation possible.

Further reading

Bateson, G. (1962) (editor) *Perceval's Narrative: A Patient's Account of His Psychosis 1830–1832*. London: Hogarth Press.

Goffman, E. (1961) *Asylums: Essays on the Social Situation of Mental Patients and Other Inmates.* New York: Anchor.

Scull, A. (2015) *Madness in Civilisation: From the Bible to Freud, from the Madhouse to Modern Medicine.* London: Thames & Hudson.

Taylor, B. (2014) *The Last Asylum: A Memoir of Madness in Our Times.* London: Hamish Hamilton.

3

SANE INSANITY

Mary Barnes

Mary Barnes (1923–2001) was born into a family which was to be accused by her of madness-inducing perversity. This was not because of a surfeit of malevolence but a surplus of congeniality:

> My family was abnormally nice.
>
> *Barnes in Barnes and Berke, 1973, p.14*

This alleged abnormal niceness was not a significant factor in her becoming an unremarkable patient of orthodox psychiatry, but it was a notable matter in her turning out to be the most remarkable patient of unorthodox psychiatry. The latter movement was headed-up by a psychiatrist who gained guru status for turning against his orthodox training as well as notoriety because of his remarkable persona which included traits of intellectual creativity, alcoholism, drug-taking and swinging from being nice to not being nice.

The psychiatric career of Barnes began in the 1950s when she was in her mid-thirties. What she was later to describe as her 'love–hate childhood' with her nice family was for the rest of her life to be refashioned into a convoluted hate–love affair with the regular and irregular sides of psychiatry, at first entrapped by mainstream mental medicine and later seduced by its mutinous offshoot. When the proponents of the former seemed to have forsaken her and she it, Barnes ardently pursued and was enthusiastically embraced, by the advocates of the latter. As with many affairs, and despite the eagerness of both parties to bond, the relationship may not only be distinctive but tempestuous.

According to the orthodox psychiatrists with whom Barnes was to be linked she was suffering from schizophrenia, and her nice family may or may not have contributed to its materialisation. According to some of the unorthodox medical practitioners who took a stance which became branded as 'anti-psychiatry' the jumbled emotional relationships in Barnes' nice family were indelibly complicit in what their orthodox colleagues considered as her schizophrenic disorder.

The anti-psychiatry movement came about in the 1960s in Europe and North America and persists in various guises today. However, it has never strictly been a 'movement' in the gist of having a united set of values and goals, and it is associated with a disparate group of medical and non-medical practitioners and theorists. Moreover, some of the anti-psychiatrists dissociated themselves from that or similar designations, while others have allegiances to substitute brands such as 'critical psychiatry'. The original band of loose associations over subsequent decades was to become even more amorphous with the only common thread amongst them a distaste for conventional medical notions of causes of and treatments for madness (Nasrallah, 2011; Whitely, 2012).

Muddled journey

A decade after Barnes was beginning her affair with anti-psychiatry a book was published describing the intimate and intense details of her emotional and bodily performances during the height of her period of madness in the 1960s. The book, which was titled *Mary Barnes: Two Accounts of a Journey Through Madness*, is both autobiographical and biographical having been written by Barnes and Joseph (Joe) Berke. Berke is medically trained and a psychoanalyst. He was also a collaborator of the leading exponent of the most vibrant and controversial element of the early anti-psychiatry movement. The exponent in question, also trained in medicine, is Ronald David Laing. It was Laing whom Barnes approached for help after what she saw as an abusive association with orthodox psychiatry[1] had ended, but her psychological difficulties remained. As the following quotation recounting an incident when Barnes was living in a therapeutic community (Kingsley Hall) set-up by Laing illustrates, her encounter with anti-psychiatry could be described similarly:

> I was in my nightdress. Suddenly beside myself, I ran out of the door screaming. 'I'll go to a mental hospital'. Joe [Berke] dragged me in slashed me across my face, crying in anguish: 'Oh why do you make me do this'? My nose poured with blood.
>
> *Barnes in Barnes and Berke, 1973, p.141*

Barnes describes how she cried after being struck, and that the crying was severe. She reports that her floods of tears, when abated, left her emotionally relieved and physically relaxed, helped by being hugged by Berke. She refers to Berke, not surprisingly, as a 'brute'. Brutish or not, she says that not only did she need to be hit but that on being physically abused she:

> [...]never loved Joe so much.
>
> *Barnes,* ibid

But, what had led to her becoming a patient of psychiatry and then anti-psychiatry? For Barnes her mind was mixed-up prior to gestation, possibly even conception:

> The big muddle started before I was born.
>
> *Barnes in Barnes and Berke, 1973, p.13*

Much of the detail in this chapter about Barnes's muddled journey into and through life is taken from Barnes and Berke's book. It is likely that Barnes and Berke colluded closely in the production of the book and its content as it could hardly be assembled otherwise. *Ipso facto* it is subjective as it is primarily autobiographical and when not so then it is one author writing about his/her co-author. Moreover, there are inconsistencies between and within the authors' narratives with regard to material content. For example, dates of admission into hospital by Barnes and her brother, and her employment history, do not always accord. However, the reflections of Barnes and Berke in their book are arrayed by more than just subjectivity and inaccuracy. Following the dictums of Laing's philosophy, what Berke sets out to do is to present a rigorously empathic grasp of his patient's early life if not pre-life and later life up to the point where she has passed through unorthodox psychiatric treatment for which he (heavily influenced by Laing) is the architect.

Laing's first and most famous book, *The Divided Self*, was published in 1960, five years prior to Barnes entering the group home he set up to implement his idea. Here Barnes was to supply further material for Laing and Berke's theorising by exposing more and more details of her journey through childhood. Here it was she became an experimental subject for their sort of healing. Indeed, by that time Laing had published a series of articles and book chapters as well as two further books (*Self and Others* in 1961; *Sanity, Madness, and the Family*, written with Aaron Esterson in 1964). In the second of these two books, Laing very much nailed his colours to an aetiological mast with regard to madness which implicated the performance of families, especially mothers, with the origins of schizophrenia. Moreover, Barnes had already read about Laing's thinking on madness, and the thoughts of those who had influenced Laing, before she had contacted him asking to become his patient.

Apart from his dealings with Barnes prior to her entry into Kingsley Hall, Laing had minimal therapeutic contact with her (Miller, 2004). But Barnes and Berke's accounts of a 'muddled' journey through madness can be seen as a pre-destined justification for Laing's idea of the domestically generated 'divided self'.

Bourgeois disrespectability

Reflecting on her early life Barnes tells of how on the surface each member of her family was kind to all of the others, how they were all well fed and clothed, and lived in a home which was neither cramped nor rundown. The Barnes family had the veneer of bourgeois respectability and contentment, but underneath the surface, its members were enmeshed in an emotionally brutalising holocaust (Porter, 1987).

The espoused friendliness and love was superficial Barnes claims. There were undercurrents of deep animosity and potentially fatal volatility:

> Violence and anger lurked beneath the pleasantries ... Deep down we were torn up with hatred and strife, destroying, killing each other. Our love was sour.
>
> *Barnes in Barnes and Berke, 1973, p.14*

Historian Catherine Arnold (2008) remarks, that Barnes' parents deserve sympathy for their daughter's display of 'monstrous ingratitude'.

Barnes' hatred and strife were directed towards her younger brother, Peter. She is explicit in recording her wish to kill him because she was forced by their mother to care for him (nicely) when he was a baby, and while she was still very young. Her detestation, she believes, was registered by her brother, who was, she reflects, embroiled in a 'spiders-web' of fury. Peter succumbed to madness before his sister and at an earlier age. Diagnosed with schizophrenia he was placed in a mental hospital for many years where he was given insulin therapy, anti-psychotic medication and electro-convulsive-treatment. Although Peter did not spend all of his life incarcerated, Barnes tells of how he eventually died 'vegetable-like' while an in-patient.

What she claims in the Barnes and Berke book is that her brother had become a scapegoat, a functional release in a dysfunctional family. In order that the family overall could maintain its sham of sanity, he was sacrificed. This happened at a point when he was making moves to untie the emotional clinch in which he (and his sister) was held by his parents, mainly his mother. The same fate was then to befall Barnes.

When Barnes was eight her sister Ruth was born, and her sister Dorothy was born when she was 13. She indicates a passionate detestation for her brother and her sisters. However, she seems to blame only the birth of the youngest sister for triggering a faecal-fetish. This habit was to return in middle-age initially as a form of messy and malodorous re-birthing and subsequently as a matchless and menacing art-form.

Familial sexuality

Although in her early childhood Barnes hated her mother, sisters and her brother, she was to become exceedingly protective towards the latter. Her early hatreds extended to her school and herself. There was only her father who was not in the spotlight for her loathing. However, there is a troublesome aspect to her relationship with her father from the perspective of acceptable familial levels of intimacy certainly by twenty-first-century legal and moral standards in countries such as Britain. A stark account of that aspect is provided freely by Barnes. She writes about how every Saturday night she and Peter were put in the same bath and attended by their father:

> My father usually bathed us … Often I would be scratching myself, as my father tickled me between my legs, and Peter would be playing with his little cock. To us, there was nothing 'wrong' about it … I love Daddy to tickle me between my legs.
>
> *Barnes in Barnes and Berke, 1973, p.23*

Barnes appears not to be troubled by this memory of her father's touching, and she and her father seem to accept her brother's aquatic sexualised diversions. Nor does such behaviour figure in her account of why she became psychologically disturbed, nor does it in Berke's otherwise comprehensive coverage of incidents in his patient's childhood which may have resulted in her mental muddle.

However, Barnes herself does construe an interpretation which coincides with Laing and Berke's interests in psychoanalysis on another sexualised event involving her brother. She explains that one night she and her brother were alone in the family house. As she lay in her bed, her brother entered her room and announced that he had come to sleep with her. She refused to allow Peter to get into bed with her and he left the room, slamming the door behind him. This left her feeling, she recalls, very frightened as she feared her refusal could have provoked her brother into lethal revenge.

Years later, her brother visited her when she was by then installed in Kingsley Hall, Barnes refers to an admission by Peter on that visit of sexual intent by him when he had previously asked to sleep with her. He was quite explicit, she writes, about his desire to commit incest, and how he had talked of wishing at that time to fondle her body and to put his penis inside her. She then discloses her own erotic desire to commit incest with her brother when he had come to her bedroom as she found him immensely attractive. Having these feelings, she comments, terrified her and made her feel guilty. Moreover, in her retrospective probing of that event, she concludes that unconsciously it was she who had attempted to seduce him. Her self-analysis continues with another self-accusation that by refusing to allow the seduction to take its course she had castrated (metaphorically) her brother. Consequently, her shame shifts from that associated with incest to her regarding herself as selfish for not even allowing her brother to touch her breasts.

This account of the sexual connection between her and her brother is patently imbibed with Freudian concepts. That Barnes should dip into Freudian theorising to explain the dynamics of and experiences in her family is hardly surprising given her association with Berke and Laing both of whom indulged in the idea of psychoanalysis. Moreover, she had been an avid reader of psychology texts before becoming a star exhibit of anti-psychiatry, and her brother may have passed on his learning as he had studied Freud's work before becoming a regular patient of psychiatry.

Nursing career

Barnes undertook a pre-nursing course at a technical school and then became a probationer nurse at the age of 17 years. She hated nursing, she hated her superiors, and she hated what she describes as the 'nursing machine'. The latter presumably refers to the hierarchical and bureaucratic system she is likely to have experienced in clinical arenas and the rote learning of her training, all of which characterised the way nurses were trained and how the health service operated in Britain before the formation of the National Health Service and for decades afterwards (Rafferty *et al.*, 1988). She did, however, like the patients because they were 'nice' to her.

Her career in nursing, characterised by her seemingly hating everything and everyone (unless they were nice to her), couldn't and didn't become a success and she soon wandered off into midwifery, at least for a while. Then, at the age of 22 years, she embarked on a career as an army nursing sister. At this point, her brother was still resident in a mental hospital. In this capacity Barnes was sent to Egypt and then to Palestine, both having British military deployments at the end of the Second World War.

It was while in the army that she fell in love with a man about whom she gives little detail other than his first name 'Ken' and that he was in the Army Education Corps. Barnes wanted to be his wife and have his child, but her wish was not consummated. Ken was to leave the army to become a priest. Soon after he left she discovered a belief in God and tried her hand at being a nursing nun in a Welsh convent. Following this experience, she became a nurse tutor.

Silence and St. Bernard's

However, by the early 1950s, she must have been showing signs of severe madness to those with whom she worked as a tutor as she was admitted into St. Bernard's Mental Hospital, a large mental hospital in London. Here she was intermittently placed in a padded cell and at times tube-fed as well as prescribed strong sedative medication by injection. Barnes was also to be given electro-convulsive-therapy and insulin therapy which her brother had also undergone during his incarceration.

Unlike her brother, however, she was to meet a medical man who offered salvation from the regular physical methods of psychiatric treatments within mental hospitals. 'Dr Werner', the medical man in question whom she describes as a 'visiting psychiatrist', would sit with her in silence, sometimes touching her hand. This 'silence of the hands' technique, she recalls affected her deeply and was the vital ingredient to improving her mental state rather than the seclusion, feeding, drugs, insulin, electricity or just time. She improved to the point of being able to return for a few years to both nurse tutoring and nun nursing, and was able to visit her parents in South Africa in 1962 where they had emigrated temporarily.

It was Barnes' and her brother's encounters with madness and mental hospitals, and her interest in psychoanalysis, which led to her writing to Freud's daughter. The famous father was by then dead otherwise presumably she would have contacted him. Anna Freud had followed in her father's footsteps and became a psychoanalyst. Barnes asked if she could become Anna Freud's patient. She is told by Freud's daughter that the best course of action for her with regard to improving her mental state is not psychoanalysis but to continue with nursing. Barnes turns to Laing.

Laing by then is in the ascendancy as a radical theorist of madness, and his ideas have been informed by Freudian thought. He agrees to see her and her brother together at his surgery in Wimpole Street, London, where he makes a positive impression on Barnes due to his friendliness and youthfulness. The eventual outcome of this meeting – a year later – is for Barnes to be admitted to Laing's alternative asylum, the therapeutic community of Kingsley Hall.

Kingsley Hall

Kingsley Hall is a brick three-story-high building situated in East End of London. It was founded in 1915 as a 'people's house' (Koven, 2015). Mahatma Gandhi had stayed there for six months in 1931 when negotiating with the British Government over the end of colonial rule of India. In the 1960s Laing took over Kingsley Hall with the intention of using it as a centre for a form of negotiated treatment based largely on the interactions the residents have with each other and with the staff.

The use of mental institutions as 'therapeutic communities' had been inferred in the work of nineteenth-century psychiatrists Esquirol and Griesinger (see Chapter 1). This approach was made manifest at Cassel Hospital in London by the psychiatrist and psychoanalyst Thomas Main (1946), and another psychiatrist, Maxwell Jones (1953), established 'social therapy' communities in a series of settings after the Second World War. While there are differences with regard to their clientele and background philosophies or restorative styles, the quintessence of the therapeutic community's philosophy are confession, cooperation and conscientiousness. Each member of the community is encouraged to express him/herself freely and to enter into decision-making over the running of the home and is expected eventually to accept responsibility for his/her own performance and to help fellow residents to reach the same level of recovery. Moreover, equality and engagement involves both residents and staff (Campling and Haigh, 1999).

Before Barnes enters Kingsley Hall she sees another of Laing's associates, an advocate of therapeutic communities, Aaron Esterson. By then Barnes had become on occasion severely psychologically disturbed and suicidal. Esterson was to become her main clinician for a year (Miller, 2004). At times Barnes hits Esterson, a practice she was to extend to other medical practitioners while at Kingsley Hall, one of whom was to reciprocate likewise. Moreover, she is given the anti-psychotic drug chlorpromazine (Largactil) by Esterson.

Preserved power

That Esterson prescribes any drug let alone this major tranquilliser contradicts the ideals of the therapeutic community for two reasons. First, the proponents of the therapeutic community espoused opposition to physical methods of treatment (Campling and Haigh, 1999). Second, prescribing medication of any sort affirms a distinction in status between the professional and his/her patient. These psychiatrists who were supposedly against orthodoxy maintained their professional privilege of prescribing what were by then orthodox pharmaceutical preparations. This extended beyond regular anti-psychotic medication to Lysergic-acid-diethylamide (LSD) which had been used, albeit irregularly, by psychiatrists, since the 1950s and was in the 1960s still legally available on prescription in the UK but only in particular medical scenarios (Brown, 2008; Dyck, 2008).

Neither Berke nor Laing, despite declarations to the contrary, fully gave up their professional authority. Laing's promise of equality in doctor–patient relationships and democracy in in-patient facilities was in practice at best inconsistent and at worse an invention. They did not give up their medical registration – at least not willingly. This would have removed a fundamental block to patient–professional inequality, although it would not have necessarily levelled the status disparity completely.

The power of psychiatry as appraised by Miller and Rose (1986) is multifarious and therefore it would take more than mere pronouncements of parity and the sharing of domestic decisions to disinvest its members from their dominance. With reference to Barnes, Porter comments:

> The truth is that Berke and his friends [Laing and the Laingians] were unwilling or unable to interact with Mary on a footing of equality. They were in control.
>
> *Porter, 1987, p.123*

From their first meeting Barnes indicates that she was in awe of Laing. For example, she tells of how in the early part of her residency in Kingsley Hall Barnes would regularly enter his room when he was not there, leave him food and change his bed-sheets.

Disintegration and resurrection

At the time when Barnes was being treated by Esterson she was not in control of her sexuality. She had a big problem with masturbation:

> About this time I seemed to get into a very bad state with masturbation …
> It just wouldn't seem to stop … Masturbation tortured me.
>
> *Barnes in Barnes and Berke, 1973, p.75*

Adding to the practical problems of this sexual craving, her religious beliefs meant that it was construed by her as exceedingly sinful. However, this excessive auto-eroticism seemed to the Laingians[2] to fit Freud's idea about developmental snags causing later psychological problems. For Freud (1905) normal progress through childhood into adulthood demands moving through multiple stages, some of which concern auto-eroticism. When a child misses or becomes stuck at a stage then for Freud the consequence may be severe neuroticism. When Berke becomes Barnes's main therapist, what he prescribes, with the backing of Laing, is emotional disintegration and resurrection.

With their encouragement and her willing participation, deep disintegration ensues. She urinates in her bed and goes to sleep. She plays with her faeces. On one occasion she threatens to cover Laing with her excrement and believes that if she had done he would still have loved her (Laing gets squeezed by her instead). She stops eating and drinking, and on Laing's advice is fed by staff sometimes using a baby's bottle. She has temper-tantrums. She stops bathing and is on one occasion carried to the bathroom by Berke. She enjoys sitting on Berke's lap. The two play hide-and-seek with her bedclothes while she is in bed. He tickles her. He pretends to bite her nose. They hug each other, tightly.

During this return to childhood (which lasts for two years) Barnes had adopted, as far as any adult of middle years could, the regressed performance recommended by Berke and Laing which they and she believed would allow deliverance from madness. Enacting base childishness would, they all thought, unstick her.

Childish playfulness and the playing of kindly parental roles were designed and portrayed by Berke and Laing as therapeutically positive activities. Through such play, Barnes would leave behind the negativity and incongruity of her actual childhood. However, some of the most adverse and discordant elements of her real childhood were replicated in this pseudo-childhood, aspects which would appear to be far more pernicious than those her doctors had identified as having being meted out by her family. Berke let Barnes know plainly that she was at times a 'pest', and Berke hits Barnes on two occasions. Although not to the same degree she feels for him, Berke is otherwise emotionally warm towards Barnes. The juxtaposition of animosity and affection by an authority figure replicates the principal communicative contradiction identified by Laingian anti-psychiatrists as the origin of Barnes' specific madness and schizophrenia generally.

What is also imitated in Barnes's 'new family' is the Freudian Oedipal phase. Barnes admits to loving Berke as a father and also of wanting him as a husband:

> To me, at times, Joe was very strongly 'my father'. In the fantasy of my family I 'marry my father'.
>
> *Barnes in Barnes and Berke, 1973, p.165*

What is more, Barnes is very territorial about her love and discloses that she wanted to kill any rival who might intrude on her love for Berke.

Faecal art

Barnes certainly had good cause to be grateful to Berke. It was he who introduced her to what was to become her passion until death. At some point in 1965 while she was in Kingsley Hall Berke had given Barnes crayons and paper which was the beginning of another career besides that of patient for one or other of the two sides of psychiatry. Her drawings, paintings and sculptures were to gain her a reputation as a respectable artist. The media has provided numerous accounts of her art which has also has been exhibited periodically ever since.[3]

This attention on Barnes' art has tended to focus on her post-Kingsley Hall art. That is perhaps understandable as her early artistic creations comprised of smearing her faeces both on canvas and the walls of Kingsley Hall. She had a particular obsession with using her faeces to craft mammary glands. Berke duly analysed her handiwork:

> Ah, but the breasts she scrawled, dabbed, smeared, and spattered ... were not ordinary breasts. They were black and were made of her shit, so smelly that people gasped when entering a room ... They proclaimed an orgy of hate and destruction which lay lightly concealed beneath the pale skin of baby Mary.
>
> *Berke, in Barnes and Berke, 1973, p.240*

Porter (1987) is highly critical of Berke's readiness to leap into stereotypical Freudian accounts of women and their alleged mental deficits. Such out-of-date theorising on gender, argues Porter, is not consistent with Laing's later commitment to psychiatry as a liberating force for women.

The unevenness of ideas brought into and generated at Kingsley Hall, however, are legion. In particular, there was an unresolved tension between the principles of a therapeutic community and those of psychoanalysis. The former promotes equality and democracy, the latter the authority of the expert. Moreover, Laing's performance as a person was peppered with paradox.

Ronald David Laing

Laing (1927–1989) was born in Scotland. He was brought up in a working-class area of Glasgow where both the strict tenets of Calvinism and the strict governance of his mother overshadowed much of his life. Laing was academically successful at his Grammar school. He describes how he wanted to become an accomplished pianist, but a sports injury meant that he refocused his ambition to enter medical school and along the way to becoming an intellectual so that he could make a difference to the 'puzzle of human misery' (Laing quoted in Itten and Young, 2012, p.4).

Changing times

The world certainly had changed and was going to change further. Laing had been born between the World Wars and was to be conscripted into the British Royal Army Medical Corps after the Second World War. Therefore he was to encounter the dramatic revamping of social conditions globally which were to take place in the following decades. Laing (*ibid.*) mentions that by then his philosophical and political interests had become wide and reformist. As well as Freud, his reading, he claims, covered Socrates, Søren Kierkegaard and Friedrich Nietzsche and he had given lectures to the local Communist Party on Karl Marx, Vladimir Ilich Ulyanov (alias, Lenin) and Leon Trotsky. His first love was ignited, discloses Laing, because the woman in question had read Franz Kafka.

Furthermore, the Barnes, Berke and Laing associations began at a time when the social condition of the mad and psychiatry was changing appreciably. In many Western countries, the policy of incarcerating large numbers of mad people was being replaced by one of decarceration. Care in the community rather than in institutions was being enshrined in mental health legislation as well as health social care policies. Rather medical authority invariably dominating, multi-disciplinary teams were instituted which threatened to dilute that dominance. In countries such as the UK these teams ideally were to comprise of psychiatrists, psychiatric nurses, occupational therapists, social workers and clinical psychologists, with the expectation of sharing decisions if not responsibility (McCulloch *et al.*, 2000; Morrall, 2000).

At that time the power of psychiatry was also being challenged by talking therapies re-entering or entering anew the treatment arena, especially psychoanalysis, behavioural techniques and humanistic counselling. These treatments did not need to be employed by medical practitioners, and indeed some had been invented in order to avoid this being necessary. Ever since Freud the main talking therapy (psychoanalysis) gained its legitimacy from the medical profession and could only be practised in the USA by medically-trained personnel. However, counselling (specifically the 'person-centred/humanistic' variety) was devised by clinical psychologist Carl Rogers to decouple talking therapy from medical control (Morrall, 2008).

Also implicated in the menacing of mainstream mental medicine by the mid-twentieth century is the offering up from the social sciences of alternative ideas about causation and cure or reconfiguration to those which concentrate only on the individual. For example, sociologist Erving Goffman (1959; 1963) was arguing that being tagged mad meant being severely socially stigmatised. The individual's 'self' was spoiled because of how society, via psychiatry, perceived madness. He also revealed in his research into total institutions (Goffman, 1961) that the social rules of the asylum meant that if you weren't mad when you went in you had to become mad before you could be allowed to recover and then let out (see Chapter 2). Sociologist Thomas Scheff (1966) was suggesting that the label of madness applied when all other categories of social deviance have been exhausted (such as criminality). Andrew Scull's (1977; 1979) sociological critique of psychiatry had led him to postulate that it assisted the State to ensure that the structure of power in society survived disruption from deviant groups, one of which is the mad (see Chapter 2). Further evidence and theorising at that time indicated that socially stressful or disorganised situations increased rates of mental disorder as well as criminality (Merton, 1957; Faris and Dunham, 1965). More recent academic work on how society affects an individual's mental state has made an association between mental disorder and socio-economic status (Hudson, 2005; Wilkinson and Pickett, 2010; Tiikkaja *et al.*, 2013).

Normalising madness

The notion that society and the individual are inseparable is accepted by Laing and his colleagues, as it was by Freud (Bocock, 2002). But Laing is particularly exercised by effects of one element of society, the modern nuclear family. For him and his colleague David Cooper (1967; 1968), the nuclear family is divisive and dislocating.

Laing and Cooper founded the Philadelphia Association in 1965 through which about 20 therapeutic communities similar to Kingsley Hall were formed throughout England. It was Cooper who first coined the term 'anti-psychiatry' in 1967 which was long after the movement, or rather movements, had begun (Rissmiller and Rissmiller, 2006). Added to Cooper's antagonism to psychiatry is a strong leaning towards Marxism. This leads him to consider the family of mid-twentieth century capitalist countries as an indoctrinating social institution. The nuclear family for Cooper serves to pacify its members and socialise them into accepting an unequal and exploitative society. Although Laing does not adopt Cooper's Marxist fervour, he does agree that the nuclear family is a pathological social institution born of modern society. It is anthropologist Sir Edmund Leach's quotation from a BBC Reith Lecture, made at the same time as Cooper was coining the term 'anti-psychiatry', which corresponds to Laing's opinion:

> [In the nuclear family] ... there is an intensification of emotional stress between husband and wife and parents and children. The strain is greater than most of us can bear. Far from being the basis of the good society, the family, with its narrow privacy and tawdry secrets, is the source of all our discontents.
>
> *Leach, 1967*

The hub of Laing's proposition about the creation of madness within families – the 'double-bind' – had already been compiled by Gregory Bateson and his colleagues (Bateson *et al.*, 1956 – see Chapter 2). Following Laing, Berke adopts double-bind as his explanatory nexus for madness and defines it thus:

> Double binding is a means for putting another in a straightjacket of guilt
> and anxiety in order to prevent him from doing something which you
> have already told him is O.K. to do. It is a marvellous tool for driving
> someone mad.
>
> *Berke in Barnes and Berke, 1973, p.92*

Laing's innovative idea in *The Divided Self* is that Barnes, and others who eventually become diagnosed with madness (specifically schizophrenia), belonged to a mad family and the only way to survive psychologically was for her also to have to perform madly. That is, some of her deeds, views and feelings, would be perceived to be her personal abnormalities to those unfamiliar with what he interpreted as the pathological processes of her family. But here again Laing is utilising another's idea. Goffman (1961) had observed the normalising of madness in the madhouse. Laing considered the mad family to be doing the same.[4]

Pseudo-patients

Laing, however, wasn't also without influence. A famous study from the 1970s which continues to be highlighted by the critics of psychiatry (for example, Bentall, 2009a), was carried out by psychologist David Rosenhan (1973). Rosenthal's study aimed to investigate whether or not psychiatrists could tell the difference between madness and normality. That is, he wanted to assess the diagnostic certainty of psychiatric diagnosis at its most basic level. He had been inspired by a lecture given by Laing (Bentall, 2009a).

Seven seemingly sane people from a range of backgrounds, males and females, were recruited by Rosenhan. The task of the seven along with Rosenhan was to attempt to gain admission to different mental hospitals across the United States. After gaining appointments at their target hospitals each complained of hearing voices, making no mention that they were taking part in a research study. All but one were admitted with a diagnosis of schizophrenia. This diagnosis persisted despite the pseudo-patients making no further mention of any symptom of mental disorder. The only detectable oddness – which made other inmates suspicious about the validity of their madness rather than the staff – was that many were anxious and all were habitually writing notes about their experience. What their notes revealed, as had been found by Goffman (1961), was that they soon were to feel powerless and depersonalised. Those diagnosed with schizophrenia on admission were discharged with the diagnosis of 'schizophrenia in remission'. Rosenhan concluded that psychiatric classification is unreliable and that psychiatrists are therefore not good at detecting sanity.

Rosenhan was criticised for both his methods and his conclusion (Kety, 1974). The study was covert and therefore, certainly by today's standards, unethical. Sampling was not robust as only a small number of mental hospitals were selected, and only a small number of researchers used. Moreover, it is hardly surprising that telling a medical practitioner you are hearing voices may lead to some form of medical intervention. Willingly being admitted to a mental hospital and subsequently continuously writing notes can hardly be construed as normal behaviour unless the staff concerned had previous experience of journalists or social scientists 'going undercover'. If they had come across such questionable professional conduct then they may have questioned the diagnoses.

Criticism also came from the staff of a prestigious mental hospital which had not been used in the study. They claimed that they could not be fooled by pseudo-patients and that their diagnosis did not have the level of uncertainty attested by Rosenhan. In response, Rosenhan informed the staff of that hospital that he would conduct a similar study on their premises, and challenged them to spot pseudo-patients amongst new admissions. A significant minority of new admissions were identified as pseudo-patients by those psychiatrists first assessing their mental state. However, Rosenhan had sent no pseudo-patients to the hospital. Concluding again that psychiatric classification is unreliable Rosenhan trumps his caustic comment from the first study that psychiatrists are not good at detecting sanity by declaring that they are not good either at detecting insanity. What both Laing and Rosenhan are indicating is that the division between madness and normality may not merely be blurred but reversed.

But what Laing had delivered in *The Divided Self* went beyond (weak) empirical evidence about the flakiness of conventional psychiatry. From his expansive philosophical interests, Laing selects two complementary theoretical strands to support his overall stance on madness. These are existentialism and phenomenology.

Existentialism

Existentialism is a philosophy made famous by a long list of luminary social thinkers amongst whom are: Søren Kierkegaard; Fyodor Dostoevsky; Friedrich Nietzsche; Martin Heidegger; Herman Hesse; Franz Kafka; Albert Camus; Jean-Paul Sartre. What is emphasised by these thinkers is the solitariness of human existence (Cohen, 1997). We are unique and isolated, alone in our journey through life no matter how many connections we make with other people, animals or possessions. We may daydream, love, be loved, have children and pets, we may live in a large family and have hundreds of friends and work colleagues, we indulge in rampant consumerism, travel, play sports, watch television, films and DVDs as well as listen to music for hours daily, connect compulsively on electronic social media, but we cannot shake off the veracity and tragedy of our solitude.

We can try to mystify the reality of our meaningless existence by fantasising sharing, caring, procuring, texting and emailing. But, to borrow a term invented by sociologists Stanley Cohen and Laurie Taylor (1992), these are only 'escape attempts'. Ultimately we are alone. Humanity is nothing more than an infinitesimal glint of animated matter drifting pointlessly in a, or one, vast and what may be an equally pointless cosmos.

For Laing (1960) many people unconsciously detect their pointlessness and this furnishes, he suggests, a psychological state he describes as 'ontological insecurity'. Ontology is the study of how we know what we are as humans, what sense we make of our 'being' in the sense of being alive and being the person we think we are. The meaning (or '*verstehen*': Weber, 1947) we make about and for ourselves is perpetually exposed to contradictory data. Mostly the messages which challenge who we think we are, are slight and our assumed self-identity is maintained or only altered marginally. However, when a loved one dies, if we lose our job or retire from the world of work, when we are diagnosed with disabling or terminal disease, fail an exam, get married, give birth, rear children, get divorced, we may have to re-adjust drastically our previous self-identity. For Laing, any in-born ontological insecurity is made much worse by certain social institutions and systems. The nuclear family and capitalism were especially capable of furnishing intense ontological angst (Laing and Cooper, 1964; Laing and Esterson, 1964; Laing, 1967; 1969).

The apparent pointlessness, inexplicability and insecurity of our existence doesn't necessarily have to descend into nihilism. Rather than becoming disconsolate, cynical and suicidal about our empty and anarchic actuality, existential psychotherapists suggest that humans can choose to make meaning from and in their lives. An individual can, given that there are no overwhelming circumstances, have the freedom to be whom and what he/she wants to be and thereby gain direction and satisfaction (Aho, 2014).

However, the realisation of and responsibility for our own personal freedom, juxtaposed with awareness of the futility of everybody and everything, may force the emergence of latent ontological insecurity or magnify what is already present. Existential philosopher Jean-Paul Sartre describes the sickening and dizzying feeling of anxiety associated with ontological insecurity as '*La Nausée*' (the nausea). While sitting in a municipal park somewhere in France, Antoine Rochentin, the focal character Sartre's novel *La Nausée*, exclaims:

> Everything is gratuitous, that park, this, town, myself. When you realise that, it turns your stomach over and everything starts floating about … that is the Nausea.
>
> *Sartre, 1965 – first published 1938, p.188*

For Sartre, existence is absurd but isn't experienced as such because we habitually hide the ridiculousness of life from ourselves. The attempt to escape reality, of course, is made all the harder because of the insight of existentialism.

Phenomenology

Conceived by the philosopher Edmund Husserl (1970), phenomenology has theoretic bonds with existentialism. For the phenomenologist, as with the existentialist, there is nothing in the social or natural world, on Earth, anywhere in the universe which has any meaning apart from that which is given to it via human consciousness. That is, nothing exists without it being perceived consciously as existing. Without consciousness, nothing can be observed, comprehended, described and then labelled. Our world is what we make of it and each one of us makes a world for ourselves.

Researchers adopting a phenomenological approach and its offshoot 'interpretative phenomenological analysis', reject notions of neutrality, tightly-conducted methods such as laboratory experiments and randomised trials, tightly systematised samples and statistical techniques to evaluate data. What they do instead is to attempt to find a high quality of meaning from their research subjects, who may be small in numbers – possibly only one (Moustakas, 1994; Smith, 2009). Interviewing an informant in-depth and at length about the sense he/she makes of his/her life or one aspect of that life is a prime technique. Accepting that meaning as a legitimate interpretation is core to phenomenological research. What an individual experiences and what sense he/she makes of that experience also is a stance taken by humanistic as well as existential psychotherapists (Wachtel and Stanley, 1997). This is in contrast to the cognitive-behavioural and psychoanalytic (and psychodynamic) psychotherapy whose practitioners are disposed to re-adjust the point of view of their clients (Morrall, 2008).

The cross-over between existentialism and phenomenology is implied in what has become the well-known philosophical axiom attributed to the Enlightenment philosopher René Descartes (1637; 1644), *Cogito ergo sum* (I think therefore I am). The notion that without conscious thought the reality of human existence and that of anything else is impossible, however, was expressed by the ancient Greek philosophers Plato and Aristotle centuries beforehand. Sartre also has a version of this sentiment that nothing exists including 'me' unless and until its existence is conceived through thought, but which includes the nauseous consequence of such thinking:

> I am, I exist, I think therefore I am; I am because I think ... [W]hy do think? I don't want to think anymore, I am because I think that I don't want to be, I think that I ... [gap in original] because ... [gap in original] Ugh!
> *Sartre, 1965 – first published 1938, p.146*

Double-bind pursuit

What all this adds up to for Laing, as had already been proposed by Bateson with his collaborators (Bateson *et al.*, 1956), is that doctors should listen to their patients and not only hear what is being said but take what they are being told seriously. Rather than attempting to objectively seek signs of a pre-formulated and scientifically verified disorder, the clinician should take as valid and substantive the patient's subjective perspective. The specialness of this perspective, argued Laing, will require special responses and Laing was certainly adept at catering for that requirement.

Laing listened to families with a member who was schizophrenic and to his patients (Laing, 1960; Laing and Esterson, 1964). From these exercises in listening he believed he heard messages which indicated the roots of ontological insecurity in the childhood experiences of the person assigned schizophrenic.

An absence of mother–child bonding and especially the lack of love and the mother addressing her own needs at the expense of her child's, are significant factors in bringing about a later intense feeling of vulnerability. Furthermore, the mother may make conditions when offering her love which are primarily in her interests, not the child's. For example, exaggerated love expressed by the mother towards her child may be a substitute for an absence of affection from and/or to an adult partner. This conditional love induces anxiety in the child which could later lead to full-blown ontological insecurity. Certain forms of conditional love have the effect of creating double-binds for the child.

Learning to live insecurely and learning to adjust to the mother's manipulations can eventually, argues Laing, lead to what conventional psychiatrists describe as schizophrenia but what he wants to understand as a rational way for the child to deal with an irrational situation. The child's 'self' in this situation has become divided. There is a mostly submerged and precarious authentic self, but also a false self he/she employs to cope with the mad circumstances in which he/she is embroiled. Eventually, the coping strategy of splitting the self cannot be maintained, the strain becomes too great and by then the genuine side is no longer intact and therefore cannot be called upon to support adulthood and survival away from his/her family. Following the splitting into two, the self may disintegrate into many discordant parts. It is at that point insanity in is likely to be diagnosed.

Predetermined guilt

What Laing displays in his writings, teachings, and interpersonal interactions at Kingsley Hall (for the latter see, for example, Robinson, 1972), however, is also a multi-divided 'self'. In particular, his existential-phenomenological self is in tension with his explanatory self. That is, if the starting point of Laing's philosophy is to give full and uncritical credence to the patient's story and meanings as presented by him/her then why does Laing then provide a particular, complicated and expert opinion on that story and on the meanings given by the patient?

By the time Barnes entered Kingsley Hall (in 1964) Laing already had a premise to prove and a message to market, a preselected prism through which to eye her early and extant performance. What he was 'hearing' was not evidence to support her perspective but to substantiate his. Years before meeting Barnes he had (in *The Divided Self*: Laing, 1960) compiled his notion of ontological insecurity, rejected madness as 'illness', and pinpointed the family as a key causative agency for what his conventional colleagues dubbed 'schizophrenia'. This discrepancy Laing passed on to Berke:

Long before I ever heard of Mary Barnes, I had begun to realize that what is commonly called 'mental illness' is not an 'illness' ... but an example of emotional suffering brought about by a disturbance in a whole field of social relationships, in the first place, the family.

Berke in Barnes and Berke, 1973, pp.83–84

Parents and in particular mothers were held responsible for the ontological insecurity of their offspring, and evidence was sought from them to confirm their culpability. Berke arranged on several occasions to interview Barnes's parents. On one occasion, and this time outside the formal set-up of a clinical conference between physical and family, Barnes' parents unwittingly supply Berke with damning confirmation of their deduced culpability. Returning from South Africa, Barnes' parents visit Kingsley Hall, but Barnes is reticent about seeing them and there is an unplanned discussion between them with Berke in attendance. Berke recalls that Barnes's mother does not show any overt anger at her daughter's lack of enthusiasm about seeing her parents after they have travelled thousands of miles to see her. But Berke reckons there were covert messages of fury wrapped-up in the mother's expression of debility which impacted on Barnes and which typified the distorted communicative patterns which lead to schizophrenia:

No mention of annoyance crossed her lips. Instead she said 'Oh, I do feel ill'. This reply immediately induced intense guilt in Mary, ostensibly for not being hospitable towards her parents. It is a manoeuvre which is typically seen in families of 'schizophrenics'.

Berke in Barnes and Berke, 1973, p.244

In the court of Laingian acuity the parents had become informants against themselves at their own trial. The victim, their daughter, was the only prosecution witness. This witness had already a prejudicial tie to the judge and to his way of thinking. Against the tenets of most judicial processes the accused were never cautioned that their answers were to be used in evidence against them, and nor were the alleged offences ever fully elucidated in their presence. The parents were entrapped.

Apart from laying claim to existential-phenomenology Berke is particularly fond of psychoanalytical precepts and Laing's quirky construal of Freud's symbols of insanity:

Eating was equated with [sexual] intercourse, and the end product of this intercourse, her excrement, was experienced as magic babies.

Berke in Barnes and Berke, 1973, p.274

Years later Barnes, when co-writing with Berke, records the characteristics of her madness in a manner which fits Freudian-Laingian phraseology:

> I didn't know then, I do now, that what I was trying to do was to get back inside my Mother, to be re-born, to come up again, straight, and clear of all the mess.
>
> *Barnes in Barnes and Berke, 1973, p.13*

The person who was to become the *cause célèbre* for an existential-phenomenological study of madness, that is Barnes, was herself already swayed by Laing's views but her stay in Kingsley Hall and long-term involvement with Berke intensified her attachment to them and their conjectural prism. She was a self-selected case study for a favoured idea generated by those who then, with her full connivance, became the embodiment and verifier of that idea.

Intellectual insecurity

Laing's evidence came from his own clinical observations and from a limited number of case studies which he selected. Further evidence was sought by Laing and the Laingians from the performance of their patients at Kingsley Hall, again comprising of a small sample considering the pool of people with a diagnosis of schizophrenia – currently 21 million diagnosed worldwide (WHO, 2016). It would seem that little if any effort was made to offer differential diagnoses or to test relevant null hypotheses such as 'there is no connection between Barnes' family background and her schizophrenia', both regular procedures in medical science.

Laing's imagination conjured-up insanity as sanity given the insane social and physical environment which the supposed insane person inhabited. Laing further considered insanity as a healing and enriching experience if a nurturing social and physical environment could be fashioned. But how can insanity be both a rational response to an irrational situation and a remedy?

Moreover, key to Laing's position on the cause of schizophrenia is the pathological character of the nuclear family within modern society. Barnes's family is far from being exceptional for the Laingians, it was exemplary. But why then does this inherent structural element of modern society not produce much higher levels of this form of madness? There is dispute over the consistency of incidence and prevalence of schizophrenia historically and cross-culturally, but this is not focused on the specific composition and character of communication within families (Os and Kapur, 2009). With regard to the societal make-up of developed countries, socio-economic status, ethnicity, age, and gender, are more relevant causative factors (Cockerham, 2013).

There have been attempts to unearth and underscore Laing's sociological imagination, particularly drawing attention to his interest in what individuals' state is the meaning of their everyday performance, what Max Weber (1947), refers to as '*verstehen*' (Howarth-Williams, 1977; Scott and Thorpe, 2006). However, Laing's claim that mothers, the nuclear family, and the economic foundation of the Western world were culpable with regard to madness requires a theory beyond that of existential-phenomenology.

Laing (1967) did profess a political position which resonates with Marx's early theorising about the way in which the capitalist economic system of economic production during the nineteenth century alienated people from many areas of their life, particularly their work (Marx, 1844/1932). For Laing, the 'normal' person had by the mid-twentieth century under capitalism become a shrivelled fragment of what he/she had the potential to become. Individuals are alienated from themselves and from each other. The mad person has become exceptionally estranged from both him/herself, others, as well as society. Personal strife is, for Laing, wedded to political strife (1967). For example, he regarded paranoid delusions not as indications of psychotic disorder but as a reasonable reaction to a persecutory social hierarchy. Madness for Laing, therefore, was at some level a fight by the individual against social oppression and a struggle for personal freedom. Psychiatry, contends Laing, should not be consumed by scientific concerns, especially those which imply only individual pathology but leading the fight against oppression and for freedom. It certainly should not, argues Laing, be reinforcing the status quo by acting as an agency of social control.

Cooper (1968), while not forgetting the individual, was more concerned with Marx's later work, his analysis of social structure and tactics for and predictions of profound social change (Marx, 1867). Cooper wanted to change the world and used the language of revolution and searched for examples of revolutionary fervour and accomplishments in South America. For him, the intelligentsia, including the anti-psychiatrists, could and should have an active part to play in replacing capitalism and tackling social injustice internationally.

But, none of the Laingians were able to successfully synthesise their theorising in order to bridge the gap between social structure, the family and the performance of individuals. Nor did their dalliance with Marxism bind them to its practical implications.

With regard to pragmatism, the Italian psychiatrist and neurologist Franco Basaglia (1924–1980) was able to successfully install profound and long-term change to the care of the mad in his country. Basaglia (1964) was influenced by existentialist and phenomenological theorists and the thoughts of Foucault (see Chapter 1) and Goffman's study of 'total institutions' (see Chapter 2). He combined ideas from these theorists, especially those which concerned power in society and that of psychiatry, and how madness is controlled (Alvise, 2013). Basaglia started campaigning in the 1960s for the replacement of the large mental hospitals. By the end of the 1970s, a new mental health law was passed instigating the setting-up of a comprehensive network of smaller clinics situated within the community. The consequences of this radical shift may not have been wholly positive. In particular, once the mental hospitals closed down there was a corresponding increase in mad people entering the prison system (Buti, 2001). What is evident, however, is that Basaglia overall made a major impact:

> The bottom line is that Italy has shown in practice, for almost a quarter of a century, that it is possible to do away with the mental hospital and to

provide a nationwide system of psychiatric care according to the principles of community mental health.

Buti, 2001, p.45

Manifestly, neither Laing nor Cooper brought about the destruction of the capitalist economic system. They were not even effective in altering appreciably orthodox psychiatry let alone bringing about its destruction in Britain or anywhere else. However, as Laing became more embroiled in celebrity and alcohol, the impact of Laing on Laing was major (Miller, 2004).

Knotted repute

All humans can be considered to have not one all-embracing 'self' but variations on a theme, or with a core but coinciding with some inconsistent traits (Feist *et al.*, 2017). However, with Laing the variations and inconsistencies are marked. Similar to his intellect, Laing's temperament was fertile yet tangled and split. Loquaciousness, amiability and compassion, coalesced with the use of hard drugs and especially hard drinking. His descent into drunkenness with many of the concomitant anti-social-behaviours associated with alcoholism strained his family relationships (Miller, 2004; Laing, 1997).

Kingsley Hall also became knotted, degenerating into tensions with patent parallels to the social situations it had been designed to surmount. Factionalism broke-out amongst the staff and some patients became – notably Barnes – once again scapegoats. Berke reflects on this irony:

> How strange that a group of people devoted to de-mystifying the social transactions of disturbed families should revert to behaving like one.
>
> *Berke in Barnes and Berke, 1973, p.262*

The crucible of Laing's social experimentation was to close in May 1970. After leaving Kinsley Hall, Barnes occupied herself writing, lecturing and painting, truly a life well-spent, and presumably a testimonial to Laing's experiment although what might have happened if she had never met Laing is beyond conjecture. When Kingsley Hall shut as a centre of Laingian experimentation, according to the historian Catherine Arnold (2008), it (again?) became a playground for a multitude of questionable practitioners and practices.

It is difficult to assess how much benefit Mary Barnes gained from her association with Laing and Berke, and from living in Kingsley Hall with any degree of objectivity particularly as subjectivity is primary to the ethos of these existential-phenomenologists and of that therapeutic community. Tony O'Brien is a nurse and tutor as had been Barnes. In his review of the Barnes and Berke book his estimation about the success of the Laingian input on Barnes' mental state contains a Laingian-style twist:

Mary Barnes was never cured. Perhaps she was never ill.

O'Brien, 2005

Can Laing retrospectively be considered to be a product of his time, his views a necessary adjustment to the rising power of psychiatry? Theodor Itten, psychotherapist, clinical psychologist and former apprentice of Laing, and body-psychotherapist Courtenay Young have marked the half-century since the publication of *The Divided Self* by Laing (Itten and Young, 2012). The contributors to Itten and Young's commemorative text, all of whom either knew him or were influenced by him, provide compliments and condemnations. The juxtaposition of intellectuality, amiability and sensitivity, with vanity, aggression and addiction, paint a picture of a fragmented character. But then he had come to fame at a point when the Western world was fragmenting and he had been raised in a fragmented family. The old world of stringent social division, sexual repression and gender subjugation, colonial rule and military might, was sitting alongside an array of counter-cultures, carnal exploration, women's emancipation, decolonisation, anti-war and anti-racist demonstrations.

From a sociological structuralist standpoint, far from being a singular and unique thinker, Laing's thinking is the product of these social strains. He has not a free mind and nor has anyone else as society (as well as neurology: see Chapter 5) constrains but also compels our ideas. From the point of view of Henry Nasrallah (2011), psychiatrist and specialist in the neurobiology and psychopharmacology of schizophrenia, past and present criticism of his profession should be welcomed. For Nasrallah psychiatry's antagonists (including Laing) operate as an incentive for maintaining professional integrity and the accumulation of scientific evidence.

Laing, and his associates thought that they could demystify reality and raise the consciousness of his patients about the reality of their sanity–insanity. Such thinking not only exemplifies immense egotism buts fits with the mid-twentieth century reification of the 'self', divided or not, as the locus of cultural adulation. Material possession, commodification and consumerism, and personal improvement, and psychotherapy are features of this 'me' society, as is personal discontent (Twenge, 2014). To borrow a phrase of journalist Rod Liddle (2014) we have become 'selfish, whining, monkeys' (see Chapter 4).

Life for Laing after Kingsley Hall, however, was in other respects to deteriorate. Laing seemingly had financial difficulties which meant that he had to exploit further his celebrity status. Furthermore, his unpredictable temper and alcohol dependency became more unrestrained. It was only towards the very end of his life that his ruptured persona showed signs of fusing with a mellowing of his mood and him abstaining from boozing (Itten in Itten and Young, 2012).

Laing's reputational legacy is one of visionary and a renegade in his profession and charisma and calamity in his personality. Such a mix means he continues to attract the attention of the media, academics and film-makers (Patton, 2015; Lawson, 2016; Mullan, 2017).

Thomas Szasz

Thomas Szasz (1920–2012) trained in both psychoanalysis and medicine. Born in Hungary he immigrated to the USA in his late teens. He was to become a long-standing Professor of Psychiatry at the State University of New York Upstate Medical University in Syracuse, New York (Schaler, 2012). Szasz was also a prolific promoter of his idea that there wasn't such a medical entity as mental disorder/illness.

Szasz is frequently described like Laing as an anti-psychiatrist (see, for example, Ralley, 2012). But like Laing, he didn't appreciate that portrayal of him and his views. Both were medically trained and had an interest in psychoanalysis. Also, like Laing, Szasz is against the institution of (conventional) psychiatry. However, unlike Laing, Szasz was not hostile to the scientific search for mental pathology in the individual. Szasz's attitude towards Laing was, however, hostile. Furthermore, he was hostile towards psychiatry whether of the conventional or unconventional variety.

Metaphors and problems

Szasz published first an article (Szasz, 1960) and then a book (Szasz, 1961) both with the title *The Myth of Mental Illness*. Following those publications and for more than 50 years afterwards, he maintained that the idea of mental illness construed as a disease of the mind is a myth. Disease, in the medical sense, affects only the body and hence the concept of 'mental illness' (or mental disorder) is oxymoronic. That is, the term 'mental' refers to an abstract or unknowable state whereas the term 'illness', as used in medicine practice, implies a concrete and identifiable condition. Therefore these two elements are mutually exclusive. What 'mental illness' becomes is a metaphorical term describing metaphorical forms.

Szasz's idea that madness is metaphorical not medical had an exclusionary clause. Some madnesses were medical, not mythical. These were those with identifiable biological (genetic, neuroanatomical, neurochemical) faults affecting the brain.

What then is the purpose of psychiatry in society for Szasz? Szsasz provides a conspiratorial version of the function of psychiatry in society and the benefits for this medical sub-discipline. The medicalising of madness, argues Szsasz provides power for psychiatry and, as suggested by Scull (1977; 1979), it controls social deviants on behalf of the State. The collusion between psychiatry and the State is akin, Szasz (1970) argues, to the Spanish Inquisition which was instigated in the fifteenth century by Spanish monarchs with the collusion of the Catholic Church. Nobody expects modern psychiatry to act like the medieval Spanish Inquisition, but underneath the surface of assumed authoritative diagnoses and treatments the profession of medicine is adjudicating over people's reactions to routine predicaments with similar fervour as religious zealots looking for signs of improper or absent faith. There needs to be, argues Szsasz, a separation of the State from the medical profession and a reaffirming of the biological (and scientific) foundation of medical practice where the mind and brain are concerned.

Supposed medical disorders such as anxiety, depression, attention-deficit, psychopathy, schizophrenia and manic-depression, are symbols dreamed-up by psychiatrists for what Szasz says are 'problems with living' (Szasz, 1960; 1961). That is, they are intangible representations of regular and irregular difficulties faced by humans in their interpersonal relationships, employment, finances, and growing up and growing old. Being born, being alive, and heading for death, inevitably manifest a matrix of major and minor plights with which humans have to contend. That psychiatry has the answers to these personal troubles is illusory.

What psychiatry is actually doing is targeting work for itself as well as acting as an agency of social control, and the consequence is that individuals lose their ability to deal with the everyday issues of their life. Medical practitioners, Szasz contends, should stay away from these problems in living and only deal with conditions that have an identifiable organic origin.

Fallacy and resolution

The fallacy of most of mental illness/disorder and the falsity of psychiatry is underscored, suggests Szasz, by fabricated psychiatric diagnostic classifications (1970; 1993; 1998). The diagnostic appellations attributed to wide-ranging aspects of human performance in the main do not have and are unlikely ever to have, any linkage to tangible disease. They are produced through a consensus by a panel of psychiatric experts who decide whether a problem in human performance is a mental disorder. That is, it is opinion rather than the empirical observation of pathology that counts as evidence in psychiatry for what is the bedrock of the whole edifice of mental doctoring. Therefore, for Szsaz psychiatry is a pseudo-science as well as a mendacious sub-division of the profession of medicine.

Some disorders listed in the various versions of the Diagnostic and Statistical Manual of Mental Disorders (DSM) and International Statistical Classification of Diseases (ICD) do have, accepts Szasz, known biological causation (for example, toxic states, senile dementia and general paralysis of the insane). But, points out Szasz, most mental disorders are not and he predicts will never be, linked to organic dysfunction. That much of contemporary psychiatric research seeks to link biological faults to, for example, schizophrenia and manic-depression, remains and is likely to remain, a fruitless endeavour (Szasz, 2010a).

Crucially for consistency in this contention of Szasz's is that if biological fault is proven, this does not mean schizophrenia and manic-depression will thereby become authentic mental disorders. He reasons that if there is a recognisable organic malfunction in the brain then it is to the neurologists that the patient should be referred. For Szsaz, neurologists, not psychiatrists or even neuro-psychiatrists and certainly not anti-psychiatrists such as Laing, provide legitimate medical authority with regard to brain disorders. Therefore, Szasz's line of argument means that schizophrenia and manic-depression become neurological disorders (Aftab, 2014).

So, for Szasz (1961; 1970; 1994) the State and the medical profession should be stripped of their conjoint role overseeing problems with living. Governments and medical practitioners ought to leave misery, agitation, odd and imaginary thoughts and excessive behaviours, to be just accepted or tackled by those whose problems they are and maybe their friends and families. Alternatively, interventions by non-medical disciplines should be sought. That is, people who have problems in living which need attention, should if they and their nearest-and-dearest can't resolve them, hire lawyers or psychotherapists to help. If the problem concerns danger to others then the involuntary intervention of the criminal justice system may be required, but in such circumstances 'madness' should not displace 'badness' as a defence for personal actions. In particular, madness in mitigation for murder or manslaughter should not be available (Szasz, 2003). Suicide is a matter of personal choice (Szasz, 1986).

What Szsaz misses in his comparison of mental medicine with physical medicine is that the same argument he puts forward about madness and metaphor can be applied to physical illnesses. Diabetes, cancer, heart disease, influenza, and HIV/AIDS, all have degrees of metaphorical representation. For example, HIV/AIDs has been referred to as a 'plague' and deserved 'punishment' for risky behaviour (Sontag, 1989).

Szasz (2010b) refers to how all medical fields other than that of psychiatry use knowledge and skills which rely on tangible diagnostic tests, interventions and measurements of efficacy. In comparison with psychiatrists, physicians, surgeons, and anaesthetists observe and test for definite signs and symptoms, provide well-tried treatments and can measure with plausible accuracy the efficacy of their interventions. However, as social thinker and Catholic Priest Ivan Illich (1975) pointed out as far back as the 1970s, the process of medicalisation has resulted in a vast number of both mental and physical disorders being made-up. Moreover, medical practitioner Ben Goldacre (2009; 2012) shows that many technologies and remedies used in physical medicine are underpinned by flaky research and dubious connections with commercial corporations.

Libertarianism

Scull (2011; 2015) castigates Szasz for his promotion of the notion that madness, for the most part, is a myth and the social constructionists for postulating that madness is manufactured. For Scull, the manifestations of madness, the meanings attached to madness, and the ways in which madness is managed, are undoubtedly shaped by the social and historical context in which they occur. Amongst the mad, points out Scull, is to be found intense suffering which cannot be deemed constructed or mythical.

Scull and Szasz also have political positions which are diametrically opposed. Scull has regularly embraced a Marxist position in his abiding critique of psychiatry although this is not so apparent of late (see Scull 2015) whereas Szasz is a staunch libertarian. Both want the social control function of psychiatry to be amputated, but Szasz, unlike Scull, wants the State's role overall to be curtailed. People need to take responsibility for their own performance, their thoughts, emotions, and behaviour, argues Szsaz. Innocent individuals should not face forcible incarceration by an arm of the medical profession. This for him is 'psychiatric slavery' (Szasz, 2010b). If people transgress social mores then that is their choice. If they transgress the law then that is also their choice and the police then have the choice to prosecute.

As with existentialism, freedom to choose is central to libertarianism, and individuals make moral choices. From this perspective, socialistic societies diminish the potential for individual progress. Also, the sociological (structuralist) notion that poor social and physical environmental circumstances hamper greatly if not prevent such progress is rejected (Otterson, 2014). Moreover, the neuroscientific position as denoted in, for example, neurolaw (see Chapter 1), which regards the human brain as beyond all or much conscious control, is countered by cognitive neuroscientist Joaquin Fuster (2013). He argues that a function of the cerebral cortex is to allow freedom to make decisions and operate self-control. Fuster, however, also recognises that the brain has a reciprocal interaction with the social and physical environment whereas staunch individualists such as Szasz pay minimal attention to the effects of environmental factors.

Celebrity and wrestling

Szasz's opinions about madness and psychiatry do not necessary jar, however, with those of Laing given that both were interested in human liberty although their purported political allegiances were different. However, Szasz shows distinct dislike for Laing as a person and towards many of his associates.

Laing and his followers are accused by Szasz (1976a; 2003; 2008; 2010b) of extreme excess and manifold hypocrisy. They were, says Szasz, recklessly negligent frauds and deceivers. In this accusation, Szasz is not alone. For example, David Abrahamson (2012) reveals discrepancies in Laing's version of what he found and what he did when he worked at Gartnavel Royal Mental Hospital as a medical registrar from 1953 to 1955. It was Laing's account of his experiences and successes with treating long-stay patients at this hospital which propelled him into the limelight as a radical thinker and gave substance to his celebrated book *The Divided Self*. Abrahamson suggests that Laing's miscommunications about what really happened at Gartnavel fit into a pattern of selective coverage on his military medical service and other aspects of his early clinical work.

A fundamental criticism by Szsaz (2010b) of Laing and the Laingians is that they misused their professional power, and despite their protestations about the evil of coercion being used by conventional psychiatrists they did themselves insist at least on one occasion that a patient was detained involuntarily. Rather than debunking the beliefs and extricating themselves from the practices of their conventional colleagues they accepted madness (especially schizophrenia and manic-depression) as medical categories and prescribed medication. They did not become 'non-doctors' or 'ex-therapists' which would have been a necessary first step to achieving their acclaimed goal of equality with patients. This quote from a resident (Dorothee) at Kingley Hall between1966–1967 reveals how Laing was pivotal to the running of this community supposedly based on parity:

> When Ronnie left that was when the disaster hit, because Ronnie [was] a magician, a shaman and an incredible being. It was a total downer. Ronnie was holding the place together. Such a place can't exist without such a key figure, it can't.
>
> *Dorothee quoted in O'Hagan, 2012*

Laing had a powerful personality and he maintained the privileges and prestige provided through membership of a powerful profession.

According to Szasz (2010b), liberation from the shackles of conventional psychiatry could therefore not be found in Laing's anti-psychiatry. Laing and the Laingians were not 'anti' psychiatry but an aberrant offshoot of it. Their 'politics of experience' (the title of Laing's book published during the Kingsley Hall period) was not radicalism but an insidious version of professional dominance and social control. Moreover, for Szasz, Laing's left-leaning politics, although less so than Scull's, are a threat to human liberty as they increase the likelihood of State involvement not only in the running of the economy but in the personal lives of everyone.

Celebrity was sought by Laing not equivalence with his patients. At the height of his fame, he appeared regularly in the media and was courted by other luminaries. Another resident of Kingsley Hall, Francis, recalls a visit from the actor Sean Connery, like Laing a Scot, who had become a famous film actor by then because of his role in the James Bond films. No matter how celebrated they had both become, they still, it would seem, required a public ego-boosting display:

> He [Connery] came to a party with Ronnie, and the two of them started Indian wrestling while we stood around and drank. They went on and on wrestling each other in the games room. They decided to see which one was tougher – James Bond or Ronald Laing.
>
> *Francis, quoted in O'Hagan, 2012*

Eventually, Szasz suggests, Laing squandered fame, family, his standing as an innovative thinker, and his professional credentials as a medical practitioner, through abusing alcohol and people. Laing was a con-man as an anti-psychiatrist and negligent as a doctor reports Szsaz (2010b). Francis remembers how he attempted suicide from the roof of Kingsley Hall, which was unsuccessful because he landed amongst junk which left him with a fracture of the spine rather than leaving him dead. He also recalls the ease of access to psychedelic preparations at Kingsley Hall:

> Ronnie used to keep acid [LSD] in his fridge… [A]nd he wasn't shy about sharing it around. He believed it was a kind of spiritual laxative, which I think is probably quite an accurate description of it. And I do remember him handing it to me.
>
> *Francis, quoted in O'Hagan, 2012*

It was, however, 20 years after Francis fell off the roof of Kingsley Hall that Laing's performance as a practitioner was to be seriously questioned by the medical authorities. In 1987 one of his patients accused him of being drunk and of physical assault. Although the complaint was later withdrawn he was forced to remove his name from the General Medical Council's medical register (Day *et al.*, 2008).

As for Barnes, Szasz (1976a) regards her as participating in Laing's charade, allowing herself to become his and Berke's chief exhibit, used as propaganda to endorse his brand of mental mending and thereby massage his reputation. As for her artwork, Szasz comments that rather than her talent having being 'discovered' at Kingsley Hall it was merely 'found'. What he seems to be implying is that 'discovery' denotes excellence whereas 'finding' does not indicate the quality of what has been located. Szasz does submit that the quality of her art has been exaggerated and observes that the painting on the cover of the Barnes and Berke book is mere finger-painting.

Adrian and Karen

There is an interesting side-issue to Szasz's assault on Laing. Laing fathered six sons and four daughters with four women. One of Laing's sons, Adrian (2010), wrote a review of Szsaz book *Antipsychiatry: Quackery Squared* where much of his anti-Laing attack takes place. In his review, Adrian Laing (who has also written a biography of his father: Laing, 1997), describes Szasz's comments on his father as 'brutal and blunt' as well as inaccurate and exaggerated. For example, Adrian Laing argues that Szasz's claim that Laing 'had no heart' was not true because he had seen his father frequently cry at the inhumanity of humans. Adrian Laing suggests that his father had more humanity than Szasz. Faced with a man who believed he was Jesus Christ, Szasz, suggests Adrian Laing, would call him a liar whereas his father would open a bottle of wine, go sit at the piano, and invite the man who though he was the son of God to 'sing and be merry'.

Laing's childhood had features of inhumanity. For example, his mother seemingly did not dispense love readily but would dispense with his toys if they had become too meaningful to him (Itten and Young, 2012). But whatever the reality of his mother's affections or how muddled Laing's memory might be of his childhood (given the muddling of his memories about other significant events in his life), he did continue to harbour great resentment towards his mother into adult life. Resentment towards him was later to surface from his family. One of Laing's daughters, who entered the same work arena as her father and became a psychotherapist, has written about his aggression towards her. Karen Laing (quoted in *Herald-Scotland*, 2009) refers to how her father generated a reign of terror in the family and assaulted her emotionally and physically attacked her in 1973 when she was 17 years old. Notwithstanding his defence of his father against Szasz's allegation of quackery, Adrian Laing is himself somewhat brutal and blunt:

> When people ask me what it was like to be RD Laing's son ... I tell them it was a crock of shit ... It was ironic that my father became well-known as a family psychiatrist ... when, in the meantime, he had nothing to do with his own family.
>
> *Adrian Laing quoted in Day et al., 2008*

Laing's legacy to himself and to his family may have been dubious, but what legacy has been left of his idea, that of Szasz's, and 'anti-psychiatry'?

Richard Bentall

There is a corresponding flourishment in psychiatric antagonism to that of psychiatric orthodoxy (regarding the latter see Chapter 5). Social-psychiatry researcher Rob Whitely (2012) suggests that this renewed wave of condemnation is as nebulous as the original set of so-called anti-psychiatrists. It includes a wide range of consumer groups, clinicians from competing disciplines, disgruntled psychiatrists and scientologists, along with social scientists and investigative journalists whose training lends to the dissembling of all and any totems of convention and authority. While some of the antagonists do make use of the ideas of their previous counterparts (particularly Laing and Szsaz) others offer novel thoughts to attend contemporary issues concerning the understanding and management of madness.

Journalist Robert Whitaker (2005; 2010) denounces psychiatry for its past ill-treatment of the mad and for its present over-reliance on what he claims are the unscientific practices of the pharmaceutical industry. The pharmaceutical industry is similarly described by anthropologist and psychotherapist James Davies (2013). Psychiatry, suggests Davies, does more harm than good and is more 'cracked' than those it is supposed to serve. For Davies, the desire for high profits of the drug companies and the yearning for elevated status and remuneration by psychiatrists mask the moot merit of medication. Mass-marketing and the misrepresentation of results from drug trials, argues Davies, hide the harm done to patients from side-effects and inadequate or misdirected treatment of their conditions. Such criticism is striking because drugs are the mainstay treatment for madness in most Western countries and making access to them easier in those in countries with yet-to-emerge and emerging economies has been recommended by the World Health Organisation (2005).

Moncrieff is a psychiatrist who contributes to this criticism about the iatrogenic upshot of the pharmaceutical industry's products by suggesting that blanket marking techniques by the industry 'woo' psychiatrists effectively because they are insecure about their status within the profession of medicine (Moncrieff and Feltham, 2013). What Moncrieff implies is that the reliance on drugs as the default treatment of many forms of madness, along with the enthusiastic embracement of vogue diagnostic technologies, draw attention, not to the strength of psychiatry's efficacy and prestige but the weakness of its occupational ego.

Psychologist Lucy Johnstone (2000) argues that the whole history of conventional psychiatry as written by its orthodox members has been misleading. For her, the medicalisation of madness since the nineteenth century has been more about professional progression through the (mis)use of power than scientific progress through valuable treatments. She challenges the position of psychiatry's fixation of biological causation by pointing to what she regards as convincing research and reasoning pointing to psychological and social factors:

> [T]here is now overwhelming evidence that people break down as a result of a complex mix of social and psychological circumstances – bereavement and loss, poverty and discrimination, trauma and abuse.
>
> *Johnstone quoted in Doward, 2013*

Richard Bentall (1956–), another psychologist, is probably the most conspicuous and erudite critic of orthodox psychiatry at present and one whose thinking amalgamates and progresses many of the ideas of past and present fellow antagonists. Bentall is Professor of Clinical Psychology at the University of Liverpool in the UK, has an academic background in philosophy as well as psychology, is a prodigious researcher, and has received awards for his clinical and scholarly activities (University of Liverpool, 2015).

Similar to Johnstone, Bentall (2003; 2009a) claims that there has been an illusion of progress. He supports the dismantling of psychiatry's diagnostic classification systems because, in his view, they are so imprecise as to be as meaningful as signs of the zodiac. He argues that the influence of the pharmaceutical corporations on psychiatry is extremely corrupting, the science used to underpin physical methods of treatment shoddy and their value largely negligible, and a fixation with biological explanation intellectually myopic and thereby not serving the interests of patients. What those professionals involved in dealing with the mad should concentrate on are the 'complaints' that the patient reports regarding his/her mental state rather than trying to fit symptoms into a 'disorder'.

Bentall is reviving Laing's (and Bateson's) missive that patients should be both listened to and heard. Bentall has a penchant for cognitive behavioural therapy as the best mechanism for inducing effective communication between therapist and patient:

> [I]f there is a cornerstone of my (broadly CBT) approach, it is respect for the patient's way of seeing the world and curiosity about what it entails. Even the oddest delusional system is the end point of the patient's honest attempt to make the best sense of the world.
>
> *Bentall, 2011*

However, Bentall (2011) diverges from the anti-science extreme views of Laing because he considers himself to be committed to empirical scientific research and to be a pragmatic clinician. Moreover, he is not portraying madness as mythical as is Szasz (unless neurological) but in need of a reconfigured understanding.

Comparing the management of madness in the developing part of the world with that in developed countries, Bentall (2011) comments that 'mental health outcomes' are similar if not better in the former. He observes that 'doing nothing' is common in the developing world. By not interfering clinically at all or only minimally with the trajectory of a person's psychological predicament other than affording social support, is an approach professionals in developed countries might adopt. The 'do nothing' (or not much) claims Bentall, could be recommended even for those who are psychotic. But, Bentall reflects, most clinicians trained in developed countries, presumably including those qualified in cognitive behavioural therapy, find interference irresistible.

Bentall and Johnstone have become advocates for an approach named 'clinical case formulation'. This approach attempts to marry what is heard from the patient with the understandings brought into the communication process by the professional, such as those arising from cognitive behavioural therapy, thereby creating a shared narrative (Johnstone and Dallos, 2006; Bentall, 2009b; Johnstone, 2014). Psychologist John Read and specialist in 'hearing voices' Jacqui Dillon, who is an honorary psychologist, campaign for fewer pharmaceutical products to be relied on in the treatment of psychoses, and for more humane psychological therapies – again cognitive behavioural therapy is favourite (Read and Dillon, 2013).

Bentall along with Johnstone, Read and Dillon, do recognise how social factors mould madness. However, the fixation with one therapy by some of those criticising those fixated with physical methods of treatment can also be criticised as being intellectually myopic particularly if the way in which society is organised has been noted as affecting madness. That is, as argued by Feltham (2007; 2014), it would seem intellectually prudent to engage in critical thinking about conceivable causes and consequences of human psychological distress which are not locatable within in the individual's psychological and biological make-up. Thereby, it would seem morally prudent to engage with therapeutic and political action to bring about social change rather than only interventions chiefly intended to bring about personal change (Morrall, 2008).

Psychiatrist Duncan Double (2006) and Moncrieff (2009) are active in developing the growing and increasingly international critical psychiatry movement which does have a wide-eyed approach to madness. They do not wholly dismiss either psychological or physical methods of treatment, but in recognition of the influence of social conditions on madness in terms of causation and recovery, they promote the use of social therapies. Critical psychiatry also advocates the diminution of psychiatry's coercive powers.

A multitude of 'survivor' groups' representing a section of patients who regard the power of psychiatry as abusive have sprung-up, some of whom have taken a lead from the professional dissenters such as Laing and Szasz. Over decades what many survivor groups have been demanding is less or no coercion, greater diagnostic accuracy, and more effective, or at least less harmful, treatments. Some survivor groups have argued for is a disengagement from, if not a dissolution of, the institution of psychiatry. Above all, they are demanding to be 'heard' (Rissmiller and Rissmiller, 2006).

Gwyneth Lewis

What therefore would a story which has been truly 'heard' existentially and phenomenologically look like? Historical and contemporary autobiographical stories of madness abound in popular literature, in magazines, academic and professional texts and journals, in news and social (electronic) media, and on the websites of mental health support and lobby groups.[5] Personal stories of madness uncontaminated by theorising, political inclination, commercial interest or the overly impassioned predetermined perspective of the author are much harder to find.

An example of a story which appears to be tamed minimally by the ideas of others or by a previous and inexorable view of the author and which reveals innovative thinking is that provided by the Welsh poet, Gwyneth Lewis. Lewis's autobiographical book *Sunbathing in the Rain* is subtitled 'a cheerful book about depression'.

Lewis submits her idea which appears as surprising to her as it may do to the readers of her book. The comments of one reader of her book, the clinical psychologist Dorothy Rowe who has researched and written extensively about depression, are reproduced on the front cover. Rowe exclaims 'Undoubtedly the best book I have ever read about one person's experience of depression'. Lewis suggests is that depression is a warning sign about the unbearableness of that person's life as it is being lived at that point.

Depression therefore for Lewis has an 'emotional logic' which does or should trigger an awareness that this feeling may have to be accepted as the start of a process of recovery but subsequently offers the opportunity to improve the quality of life. Extending that logic Rowe implies that 'feeling low' is an essential element of existence and therefore should not be prevented, expunged, feared or despised, but embraced.

Practical tips when depressed are supplied by Lewis. Examples are: don't wish for the depression to go away; don't tolerate other miserable people; and don't make major decisions while depressed such as running away or growing potatoes in the Scottish Highlands. But, Lewis dismisses the 'lies' of affirmative interventions, practical or otherwise, which emanate from positive and cognitive-behavioural psychology. That is, when psychotherapists advocate finding favourable happenings when everything happening is experienced as unfavourable, some of which are incontrovertibly misery-making such as the death of a loved one, is professionalised emotional trickery. Moreover, advocates of 'clinical case formulation' are deliberately adding their professional discernments, conspicuously those of a cognitive-behavioural hue, to what they believe they hear from their clients.

This criticism of cognitive/positive precepts connects with her favouring sympathy over empathy. The latter for Lewis is unfeasible. That is, it is impossible to gain a full understanding of another person's feelings even if it were possible for that person to understand and express his/her feelings candidly, coherently and consistently. There is too much interpretative filtering and fudging with regard to perception and transmission for both.

A further degree of communicative contamination is evident in Lewis's account of her depression and depression as an expected part of living beyond that which she highlights as occurring in certain therapies and which defies empathy. There is an obvious backdrop of medicalised madness to Lewis's account which she does not acknowledge. She refers to depression as a 'serious disease' and sought assistance from a psychiatrist. She mentions that she received wisdom from an Archbishop of Canterbury, and a concept or two of Freud's enters her story. Furthermore, such comments as Rowe's, although retrospective, are analytical. Lewis also had a previous conviction she was cursed, in her own view, because she was not a 'viable person'.

Hence, a truly 'clean' existential-phenomenological-formulated told and heard story may never be possible as the ideas of listeners (or readers) and those of the author can never be expunged fully. What sculpt those ideas further are the sways of biology and society.

Summary

In November 2000 Barnes (2000) wrote on her website a 'finale' in which she refers to having reached the age of 77 years, and how she suffers from osteoarthritis in her spine which means that if not laying on her bed she is confined once again but this time to a wheelchair rather than a padded cell. Otherwise, she writes, that she is in good mental and physical health, and enjoys the beauty of where she is living, the Highlands of Scotland (although no mention is made of potatoes). She asks whoever is reading her website to pray for her and for 'Joe' (Berke).

Berke wrote on that website an 'epilogue' the following year:

> Mary died on Friday morning, the 29th of June 2001. I had spoken with her the night before ... Mary left a rich legacy. She was a vibrant,

expressionistic painter and sculptor who inevitably used her fingers in place of a brush to great effect.

Berke, 2001

Berke comments that he believes Barnes was a 'culture hero'. Her journey into and out of madness had, in his view, resulted in her being renewed, her 'self' having been cleansed of those experiences which had led her into psychological difficulties. It had also, he asserts, confirmed Laing's idea about madness.

Twelve years later Barnes' work featured in the 'Art in Asylum' exhibition in Nottingham, October–November 2013. Berke (2013) appears in a video showing Barnes' paintings at the exhibition which is posted on a website dedicated to her. Berke and unnamed others offer evaluations on the meaning of the work, drawing specific interpretations about Barnes' madness from the paintings. Even in death, she is still being analysed. His promised 'Mary Barnes: The Movie' has to-date not materialised.

Thomas Szasz, who died in 2012, has not to-date had a film made about him. However, his books, articles and videoed lectures and interviews, continue to be widely available.

Laing died in 1989 while playing tennis in St Tropez, France. His comment immediately after suffering the heart attack which led to his death poignantly points to the double-bind of multiple contradictions and struggles in which he was trapped throughout his life, as well as to a last gasp of rebellion against his profession. As he lay on the ground of the tennis court and after being told that a doctor had been called to attend to him, he replied:

Doctor, what fucking doctor?

Laing quoted in Bentall, 2009a, p.74

At the time of writing Richard Bentall is alive. He continues to be a prodigious producer and publisher of research and thoughts.

Has the institution of psychiatry changed or is it likely to do so in any of the directions proposed by the psychiatric antagonists? How sound are the disparaging ideas of psychiatry? May psychiatry have taken a wrong epistemological path by concentrating on finding and fixing flawed biology as argued by Bentall, misguidedly following science as argued by Laing, or misdirected science as argued by Szasz? Are more of the mad 'sunbathing in the rain' in the sense meant by Lewis? In Chapter 4 the connection between the psyche and society as opposed to biology is pondered, while in Chapter 5 there is consideration of the furthering of science in psychiatry on the back of biology.

Notes

1 Where 'psychiatry or 'psychiatrists' is mentioned in this chapter without an accompanying adverb this should be taken as meaning orthodox/conventional.

2 The expression 'Laingians' is used as shorthand for Laing and his co-thinkers such as Berke and Esterson.
3 A recent example of an exhibition is the 'Mary Barnes: Boo-Bah' held at the Nunnery Gallery in London during January 2015.
4 Laing's indebtedness to Bateson's work is indicated in a series of letters between the two in the early 1960s, and he went to the USA to meet with both Bateson and Goffman (Mind For Therapy, 2016; Burston, 1996).
5 Examples of a range of singular and collected autobiographical works in the academic/professional arena are referred to in this book and examples in the popular media and distributed by lobby/support can be obtained easily through internet searching the relevant sites.

Further reading

Barnes, M., and Berke, J. (1973) *Two Accounts of A Journey Through Madness*. Harmondsworth, UK: Penguin. [First published 1971, MacGibbon and Kee, London].
Bentall, R. (2003) *Madness Explained: Psychosis and Human Nature*. London: Allen Lane.
Laing, R. D. (1960) *The Divided Self: An Existential Study in Sanity and Madness*. Harmondsworth: Penguin.
Szasz, T. S. (1972) (first published 1961) *The Myth of Mental Illness*. St. Albans: Paladin.

4

INSANE SOCIETY

Stephen Fry

Stephen Fry (1957–) is a self-confessed madman. Indeed, Fry pronounces persistently and passionately about his insanity. But there is more to Fry than madness and more to madness than the personal (biological/psychological) constituents of any individual. There is society to consider.

Troubled treasure

By his own testament, Fry is publically known in many countries including Britain, Russia, Canada, New Zealand and Australia, and his books have been published in scores of languages (Fry, 2015). He is a polymath who accepts the description of 'modern Renaissance-man', although he insists that unlike the original multifaceted men such as Michelangelo and Leonardo da Vinci, he does not wear tights (CBS, 2012).

Prince Charles considers Fry a 'national treasure' (Singh, 2010), and according to Fry, has forgiven him for snorting cocaine in Buckingham Palace (Turner, 2015). Furthermore, Fry has been cast as a fictional British Prime Minister in a television series, his views have apparently been sought by an actual Prime Minister, and in an Internet poll, he was voted the public personage most British people would want as their Prime Minister (Nissim, 2012). Fry is an actor, comedian, author, television presenter, social media aficionado, a 'popular intellectual', promoter of gay rights, mental-health activist, humanist, intermittent celibate, reformed alcohol and cocaine abuser, and ex-criminal. He has contributed hundreds of columns and articles for newspapers and magazines and has written four novels and three autobiographies – so far. He played the lead in the film *Wilde* and a First World War army officer (Melchett) in the television series Blackadder, and presented his 2008 television series *Stephen Fry in America* for which he travelled across 50 states.

But, performing for Fry has not always been without its difficulties. Whilst starring in a run of the West-end of London theatre production, *Cell Mates* he abruptly walked out which disconcerted the play's company and especially the director (Gray, 1995). Future performances had to be cancelled as Fry could not be contacted for several days. He had gone, by ferry, to Belgium. Years later Fry was to present a two-part award winning documentary for the BBC in 2006 titled: *The Secret Life of the Manic Depressive*. In this programme he makes reference to his 1995 disappearance, explaining that he had become highly agitated and suicidal. These thoughts and emotions he had first experienced when at school, but it was not until after his theatrical debacle that they were to be ascribed by him as indicative of manic-depression (Fry, 2004; 2011).

Born in London, Fry's early life was by his own estimation, troubled. He was expelled from the private school he was attending when he was 15, and from a subsequent school. Two years later Fry stole a credit card from a friend of his family, was caught, confessed and sentenced to three months in prison. When released from prison he went back to the college he had been attending prior to his short-lived criminal career and was to settle well enough into his studies there to gain a scholarship for entry into Cambridge University. Although successfully gaining a degree in English Literature, what was of greater significance to his future life as a public figure was joining the Cambridge Footlights where he met a number of other nascent celebrities including his long-standing comedic partner, Hugh Laurie (Fry, 2004; 2011).

Sexual politics

An aspect of his troubled early life was his rising awareness of his homosexuality, but which had to be both contained and kept quiet due to the prevailing homophobic attitudes (Fry, 2004; 2011). Keeping quiet about being gay is not now part of Fry's private or public way of being. Fry has become a prominent celebrity figure challenging bigotry about homosexuality in the international political domain. The prime of example of his involvement politically in this respect was his call for the boycotting of the 2014 Winter Olympics in Sochi because of alleged 'anti-gay' actions by the authorities and in particular prejudicial laws which had been newly introduced by the Russian Federation Government. In an open letter addressed to the British Prime Minister and members of the International Olympic Committee, he made an impassioned plea for cancellation. The President of the Russian Federation, Vladimir Putin, is accused of scapegoating gay and lesbian people in the way Hitler did the Jews (Fry is Jewish), the violent and sometimes fatal consequences of which Fry finds emotionally distressing:

> Every time in Russia (and it is constantly) a gay teenager is forced into suicide, a lesbian 'correctively' raped, gay men and women beaten to death

by neo-Nazi thugs while the Russian police stand idly by ... I for one, weep anew at seeing history repeat itself.

Fry, 2013

Fry entered further into sexual politics when he claimed that (heterosexual) women do not like sex and only have sex to entrap (heterosexual) men, whereas gay men demonstrably enjoy sex because they are unrestrained in their desire for casual encounters. Seemingly, feminists were flabbergasted at Fry for delving into the depths of female psychology and desire without any relevant first-hand knowledge (Vernon, 2010). A little less politically-incorrect from a feminist point of view but nevertheless somewhat inflammatory from the point of view of women generally, is Fry's oft-quoted retort when asked about when he knew he was gay:

It all began when I came out the womb. I looked back up at my mother and thought to myself, 'That's the last time I'm going up one of those'.

Fry quoted in Gordon, 2010

Towards the end of 2016 Fry had gained over 12 million followers on the Internet social media site Twitter (Twitter, 2016), and nearly 20 million 'hits' on the Internet search engine, Google (2016). His website contains his extensive Internet 'blogs', and a 'store' from which to buy his books, his audio and DVD recordings, and themed t-shirts (StephenFry.com, 2016).

Meteorological metaphor

Fry has also resolved the meaning of life and the secret of happiness, which as it turns out is to get on with it (Fry, 2014). Life is meaningless, as Fry explains and recommends making meaning out of life by living it as fully and as well as possible. His explanation and recommendation are contrary to the causative and curative precepts of orthodox psychiatry with regard to manic-depression (bipolar disorder). Fry espouses a philosophy analogous to Laing's (1960) existential-phenomenology, which has been discussed in Chapter 3.

In a recording of an interview in front of a large audience with an unidentified interviewer, Fry provides a meteorological metaphor for how the manic and the depressive aspects of manic-depression feel for him. If it's raining when out for a walk, says Fry, normal people may accept that it feels miserable now but believe that it will become sunny again on this or some future walk. The manic-depressive who is in a depression feels that the rain will be perpetual, that it will never again be sunny. When it is sunny, however, the manic-depressive in manic state may feel not only pleasure but ecstasy, and believe that it will never rain again:

It's raining, the sun will now never come out ... Life is so black ... But the fact is it will come out, and in the case of a bipolar person it won't just be normal it will then go super-normal. They will become incredibly sunny … your grandiosity knows no bounds.

Fry, 2010

Metaphor is at the heart of Szasz's (1961) idea of mental illness/disorder mostly being metaphorical, which is also discussed in Chapter 3.

It is, however, more often orthodox psychiatry's version of manic-depression (bipolar disorder) to which Fry adheres in the main when referring to his own condition, that of others, and in his mental-health campaigns (see for example: Time to Change, 2012).

Metaphor and purism

Psychiatry regards manic-depression, alongside schizophrenia, as a major mental disorder (Semple and Smyth, 2013). Manic-depression, as with schizophrenia, is included under the psychiatric rubric of psychosis. Both are thought to have genetically inherited root causes, which produce higher incidents of the disorder in particular families (Lichtenstein *et al.*, 2009). Neurochemical imbalance, which results in higher or lower levels of particular neurotransmitters such as dopamine and serotonin, is also implicated (Benes and Berretta, 2001).

Hallucinations and/or delusions are primary to the medical diagnosis of psychoses (Semple and Smyth, 2013). The manic-depressive is more liable to be deluded than hallucinatory. The form of his/her delusions will depend on whether depression or mania is being experienced. In Britain it is estimated that up to 5 per cent of the population have indications of manic-depression (Bipolar UK, 2016).

However, as it does with other mental disorders, psychiatry defines not one clearly demarcated condition but a spectrum of conditions which are considered mild at one end of the spectrum and severe at the other. The manic-depression clan of conditions in the DSM-V have been renamed 'bipolar and related disorders' and now include: bipolar I disorder, bipolar II disorder, cyclothymic disorder, 'manic-like phenomena' brought on by drug abuse, or physical medical disorder, and 'other specified bipolar and related disorders' which do not fit the aforementioned categories (American Psychiatric Association, 2013). The difference between each of these sub-categories is a matter of partial testimony by the patient and fine judgement by the diagnostician. Furthermore, what might be diagnosed as a hallucination or delusion is dependent on perception. For example, belief in God and sensing godly visitation may be venerated by the pious, doubted by the agnostic, scorned by the atheist, respected by the humanist or diagnosed as schizophrenia by the conventional psychiatrist. Opinion, however, is then dependent on other factors such as surveillance opportunities, the social setting and historical period, and especially the quantity and quality of power owned and exercised by the observer, the observed and those with substitute standpoints.

Kay Redfield Jamison (1993; 1995) is a manic-depressive who, similar to Fry, has publicised widely, details of her emotional life which as with Fry frequently fluctuates between deep misery and heightened excitement. She is also a clinical psychologist who although not trained in medicine is Professor of Psychiatry at Johns Hopkins University in the USA. What Fry and Jamison also have in common is that they both accept that they have the medical disorder of manic-depression.

Jamison is a biological purist in terms of genetic causation. Writing in the mid-1990s, Jamison (1995) refers to the results from the twin-studies and examination of incidence in families leaving her in no doubt that the gene responsible for her condition will be found. Genetic pointers for both schizophrenia and manic-depression continue to be proclaimed but as yet 'the' responsible gene for either, particularly one which excludes other biological intricacies and psycho-social factors, has not been affirmed (see Chapter 5).

Endure and embrace

Surprisingly, given that Fry and Jamison in their respective autobiographical accounts describe in detail the intense suffering they undergo with their condition, they are both equivocal about what psychiatry regards as the classic drug treatment for manic-depression – lithium (Royal College of Psychiatrists, 2016). Lithium can have severe side-effects and potentially dangerous complications, and there is the inconvenience of regular medical tests to ensure the correct levels of the drug are occurring in the blood to avoid life-threatening toxicity (Haussmann *et al.*, 2015). However, Fry and Jamison infer another reason for questioning the value of taking lithium. Manic-depression is the type of madness both Fry and Jamison profess to endure *and* embrace.

Fry fears his manic-depression, but whilst the depression is loathed the mania is prized:

> I love my condition too. It's infuriating I know, but I do get a huge buzz out of the manic side. I rely on it to give my life a sense of adventure … giving me the energy and creativity that perhaps has made my career.
>
> *Fry quoted in Owen, 2006*

Jamison (1993) is caught between the overall dread concerning her condition and its beneficial effects. She recalls the deep despair on the one hand and the intense frenzy on the other but recognises that manic-depression has given her chances in life which she otherwise would not have been offered and if offered would not have taken.

Creativity and genius

For Jamison, the bright side of her manic-depression is manifested when she is mildly manic. She believes that an elevated mood, heading towards but not reaching euphoria or superciliousness, allowed her to be more passionate in love and achieve more in her career. However, her depression has also allowed her to value fully the sunny days when they do arrive. Both she and Fry imply that had a choice been possible they would not want to have avoided being born with manic-depression or wish to have it subdued by lithium or (potentially) gene-therapy.

Such ambivalence has also been noted in some who have been diagnosed with schizophrenia. That is, hallucinations may offer insights into the psyche and the world that debilitate those who do not have such experiences. Hearing, smelling, seeing, tasting, or tingling, in unique ways can be considered positive attributes (Chadwick, 1997). Believing that you have a superior intellect, outstanding practical skills or enhanced physical attractiveness beyond what your personal history or perceived abilities would suggest, may lead to imaginative career changes, inspired quests, acts of superhuman bravery or erotic adventures. It could also lead to disappointment if not incarceration.

Fry and Jamison are patently intelligent. The former's cleverness is lauded. In 2006 Fry was voted 'Most intelligent man on television' by readers of the British magazine *Radio Times*, and in 2013 he was named 'Britain's most influential man' in a survey of 40,000 men for the Internet site AskMen.com. The question of a connection between madness and cleverness has been mooted regularly (Bean, 2008). The millions of people who are diagnosed with a serious mental disorder, who are debilitated by it and by the treatments, who live in poverty, are unemployed or unemployable, stigmatised and mistreated, and who have markedly shorter lifespans that the average, indicate that this connection is tenuous. On rare occasions physical, psychological and social deprivation, can be overcome, but disordered minds and disordered societies are in the main not conducive to intellectual virtuosity.

That there is a link between manic-depression and creativity may seem more tenable. Jamison posits emphatically a case for this link. She points out that manic-depression or depression is vastly more prevalent amongst writers, composers, poets and artists than in the general population (Jamison, 1993). Research indicating such a link is not convincing advises Professor of Psychiatry at Harvard University Albert Rothenberg (quoted in Sample, 2015). Jamison's reckoning on the matter is described by psychologist and psychotherapist Judith Schlesinger (2012) as drenched with fuzzy assertions and massive exaggerations.

Celebrity and narcissism

Fry is not only clever and creative but a consummate confessional celebrity. Whilst linking madness, cleverness and creativity may be misleading might the link between madness and celebrity be more certain? There has been an argument put forward for such a link by a range of thinkers. Some regard the seeking of celebrity as indicative of psychological pathology in the individual. For example, one author has noted what has been referred to as an 'unusual personality structure' in comedians (Ando *et al.*, 2014). Others regard both the seeking and the veneration of celebrity as a consequence of pathology in the social system. What is mentioned commonly on both sides of that debate is narcissism.

Fry, in his *More Fool Me* autobiography comments that those he describes as 'celeb [celebrity] haters' accuse 'most celebrities of being narcissists' (Fry, 2015, p.35). He accepts that this assessment may be correct. He also admits that publishing a series of accounts about his life is a narcissistic undertaking:

> So now I must consider how to present to you this third edition of my life.
> It must be confessed that this book is an act as vain and narcissistic as can
> be imagined: the *third* volume of my life story? [emphasis in the original]
>
> *Fry, 2015, p.4*

Individual full-blown selfishness has been credited as a mental disorder by psychiatrists since the mid-twentieth century. Narcissistic personality disorder has the principle symptom of a bloated sense of self-importance, extravagant attention-seeking, hyperbolic self-promotion, the airing of virtues or sins, and little or no interest in others apart from feigning curiosity in order to gain further attention. Diagnosis hinges, however, on a symptom which narcissistic personality disorder has in common with personality disorder *per se*, that is the absence of empathy (Baron-Cohen, 2011).

Christopher Lasch

Historian and social critic Christopher Lasch (1979) believed he had identified the rise of a culture of narcissism which for him had begun in the nineteenth century but had increased in intensity towards the latter part of the twentieth century. An orientation to satisfying the self rather than having commitments to and recompenses from society, community and the family, directs individuals towards programmes of self-improvement, collecting signifiers of material accumulation, personalised adorning and auto-pleasuring or one-way sexual gratification rather than mutual and enjoined copulation. Celebrity is admired and pursued as it ostensibly denotes full 'self' actualisation, a salutation to outstanding individual accomplishment.

However, much of modern celebrity is not the outcome of unprecedented personal triumph but a means of achieving social success. Successfully selling 'the self' to the masses can bestow exalted esteem, sizeable financial remuneration and concentrated if capricious public attention. Moreover, no matter how fatuous or ignominious the origin of the celebrity, it can be sustained through a diet of publicity. The self becomes fed by its own fame or infamy in a self-sustaining carnivorous cycle of corpulent conceit. Celebrity is the epitome of narcissism, and narcissism epitomises celebrity.

Marginal madness

Although Lasch accepts that narcissism is lauded and endemic in Western culture, he argues it is not normal. The psyche becomes damaged through such excessive egotism. Lasch is influenced by Freud's idea that narcissism was necessary to assist in developing the individual's understanding of his/her 'self', but socialisation normally would contain the ego's would be excesses (Freud, 1914). For Lasch, if selfishness is not contained because socialisation is pulling in the opposite direction, it is not necessarily symptomatic of full-blown personality disorder or possibly psychopathy (anti-social personality disorder). Rather it is for Lasch a 'marginal madness', more akin to what psychiatry has come to describe as 'borderline personality disorder' (Bateman and Krawitz, 2013).

However, not only is there a specific debate over the cause of personality disorder being nature or nurture, but also one over its character and margins. These two debates are accentuated with regard to psychopathy/anti-social personality disorder. James Blair and his colleagues from the Unit of Affective Cognitive Neuroscience at University College London, believe firmly in the faulty biological base of psychopathy/anti-social behaviour disorder (Blair *et al.*, 2005). But they admit that finding the precise biological cog separating nature from nurture continues to be problematic. Whilst they believe genes are responsible, which ones they are remain unidentified, as does the way in which these genes interact with anatomical areas of the brain such as the amygdala and orbital frontal cortex which are also thought to be involved. The definition of psychopathy/anti-social behaviour disorder remains moot. Despite plentiful funding, time and technology being allocated to find a clear-cut cause and effective treatment for psychopathy/anti-social behaviour disorder, neither has so far been identified.

Furthermore, there continues to be a dispute over whether anti-social personality disorder and psychopathy are indistinct or different conditions, as well as disagreement about this genus of human performance being one principally of personality, emotions, or conduct (Blair *et al.*, 2005; Andrade, 2008; Baron-Cohen, 2011). If the latter, then the question is raised as to whether or not misconduct (that is, delinquency and dangerousness) is a legitimate diagnostic domain for psychiatry rather than for the criminal justice system (Szasz, 2003).

There remains the interminable wrangle over whether or not psychopathy is synonymous with badness rather than madness (Babiak and Hare, 2006; Taylor, 2011). There are life-lasting and life-changing consequences for individuals and considerable policy implications for governments regarding the decisions made in courts concerning the divide separating evilness from mental disorder. The philosopher Mary Midgley (2001) remarks that in the last century the confusion concerning who and what can be considered wicked has increased because natural science and social science have offered justifications for mundane bellicosity and grotesque barbarity. Male aggression, domestic murder and Nazi atrocities, all have evolutionary, biochemical, social-learning and socio-environmental explanations which detract from full or any personal liability. Moreover, a common agreement on what is a normal personality remains elusive. Therefore, what a pathological personality is, what separates one type of personality pathology from another, and what is on the borderline of normality, is immeasurable unless the dubious technique of teleological reasoning is employed (see Chapter 5).

Selfish whining

Like Lasch, psychologists Jean Twenge and Keith Campbell (2009) postulate that pathological narcissism (that is, narcissistic personality disorder) is not identical to 'normal' narcissism furnished by a 'narcissistic culture'. Functionally, however, the separation of pathological narcissism for normal-narcissism is for Twenge and Campbell mainly a matter of degree. The pathological state confers higher levels of grandiosity and a very low if not a total absence of empathy, which may furnish failure in many routine activities of daily life such as maintaining mutuality in interpersonal relationships. On the other hand it may yield success in banking, business and politics. That is, normal narcissists may have a competitive edge when attempting to achieve corporate and civic senior office (Ronson, 2012). On Tuesday 8 November 2016, businessman and celebrity Donald J. Trump was elected as the President of the USA. Both before and after his election allegations appeared in the media that he suffers from 'narcissism' or more pointedly 'narcissistic personality disorder'. These presumptions regarding his temperament are made by both journalists and clinicians (for example: Gardner quoted in Alford, 2015; Barber, 2016; Rawnsley, 2016). If Trump is in any sense narcissistic, and this view remains speculative particularly as no face-to-face formal clinical assessment has either been attempted or admitted, then his election may imply as much about the culture of his country than any pathology in his personality. A culture in which narcissism has become epidemic is itself pathological according to Twenge and Campbell. When elevated narcissistic performance confers reverence, remuneration and influence, then for them the whole of the social system has become 'diseased'

Journalist Rod Liddle (2009) as with Lasch, Twenge and Campbell, looks beyond the individual to explain why narcissism appears to be prevalent. His appraisal is less academically measured and more journalistically vitriolic. He is particularly incensed with Fry. Liddle lambasts Fry for what he alleges is his elevated narcissism, and especially his infatuation with contemporary communications technology which provides him and countless others with an avenue for relentless self-indulgence.

Liddle isn't just angry with Fry and the rest of social media devotees but with Western society. Liddle associates what he regards as trivial, meaningless, hollow, narcissistic disclosures with what Twenge (2014) has called the 'me generation', those born during 1955–1985 in the West. This generation arrived when the culture of narcissism and the cult of celebrity were starting to bloom. It is, argues Liddle, absurd that so much time and effort is spent by individuals on themselves and encouraged to do so by a materialistic and individualistic culture, and yet happiness remains elusive. He points out that people in the West live longer, are materially much better off, possess vastly more tangible commodities, can access a wide range of entertainments, and take more holidays, than ever before. Besides being consummately selfish these supposedly superior primates (humans) have returned to an atavistic state and one which is accompanied by a doleful and querulous disposition. They are 'selfish whining monkeys' (Liddle, 2014).

Chic insanity

If culture foments narcissism, and if psychiatry can so readily reconsider it as mental disorder, could it be that manic-depression is also affected by culture, and could it be susceptible to similar reconsideration? Have the values and practices of today's Western society which have infiltrated much of the rest of the world (given that there is resistance by, for example, Islamicists, to Western globalisation) sponsored both an epidemic of narcissism and an upturn in the incidence of manic-depression? Furthermore, are narcissism and manic-depression culturally entwined? Has it become fashionable to be bipolar? Psychoanalytical psychotherapist Darian Leader comments on these possible connections:

> If the post-war period was called the 'age of anxiety' and the 80s and 90s the 'antidepressant era', we now live in bipolar times.
>
> *Leader, 2013*

The huge rise in medical diagnosis and self-diagnosis of manic-depression since the mid-twentieth century has in part occurred due to the nebulousness of the condition which has led to, as mentioned above, the use by psychiatry of the 'spectrum'. The spectrum serves psychiatry when faced with uncertainty (Leader, 2013). The bipolar spectrum allows for what might otherwise be taken as eccentric, moody or idiosyncratic elements of an individual's performance to be medically pigeon-holed. It has also become a trend for celebrities to accommodate such pigeon-holing to either enhance their fame or excuse their infamy (Barker and Buchanan-Barker, 2011; Whitaker, 2010; Moncrieff, 2009). Manic-depression's historical association with cerebral dexterity, including comedic ingenuity, makes it a better choice of label for offensive eccentricities, unlawful conduct, drug and alcohol abuse or a turbulent temperament, than criminality, schizophrenia or psychopathy. From the mid-twentieth century onwards, the advancement of medicalisation, a swelling of appeal and opportunity to access medical information which allows members of the laity to nominate their own disorders, a public and media with an insatiable appetite for disclosure, and easy access to and willingness to participate in mass communication, have all provided the cultural standards and openings for the hawking of self-serving narratives.

Many, perhaps most, of these self-serving narratives exemplify narcissism and embolden narcissists. A celebrity announcing to the world that he/she has a major mental disorder, or more specifically one which bears much stigma such as schizophrenia or psychopathy, will attract attention but also ignominy. If the 'choice' of madness has the hallmark of ingenuity as has manic-depression, then admiration may accompany the attention this brings. This admiration can lead to others choosing to embrace that label. Psychiatrists Diana Chan and Lester Sireling recognise that there may be an effect on the rate of manic-depression due to the celebrity claims and disclosures such as that afforded by Fry. That is, they claim to have observed in their clinical practice what they describe as a new phenomenon of 'I want to be bipolar'. They mention Fry's two-part documentary in which a range of well-known actors, singers and comedians, along with lay people, celebrate the positive aspects of the condition:

> [Nearly all of those interviewed by Fry] commented on the enjoyable experience of having new ideas with increased activity, the excitement of feeling high in mood, and powerful, and how these experiences would be difficult to relinquish. Clearly experienced as advantageous by the interviewees, evidence has shown that bipolar disorder is strongly correlated with creativity and literacy.
>
> *Chan and Sireling, 2010, p.103*

Some of their patients, they argue, are seeking a diagnosis of manic-depression to explain what might have been observed by their relatives as disconcerting behaviour, emotions or thoughts. An inference from their report on what is occurring in Chan and Sireling's clinical practice is that bipolar as a diagnosis may vindicate what otherwise might be experienced or perceived to be unacceptable elements of an individual's performance, and provide enhanced social status because of the association with celebrity.

Far from decrying manic-depression as unwarranted medicalisation, Chan and Sireling conclude that it may be underdiagnosed. Their advice to their colleagues is to be aware that there is false and real manic-depression, and they need to be skilled in separating out those whose madness is fallacious. Psychiatry has not always fared well at that task. Darian Leader (2013) also recognises that those who really do suffer because of their moods swings, rather than enjoy them need professional help. But for Leader, a more humane approach should be adopted than that of the traditional medical one – principled presumably on psychoanalysis – which respects both the individual's past and present personal stories of his/her life.

Erich Fromm

If narcissism is not a malady stemming from an individual's essence but a cultural sickness then what is at the root of a culture which turns humans into what Liddle refers to as 'selfish monkeys'? From where does that culture arise?

Defects and degradation

Some of those with ideas about insanity, for example, those sociologists who favour structuralism, accept that conventional psychiatrists, along with most psychologists and psychotherapists, are correct in claiming that there are real disorders of the mind/brain. But rather than focusing on faults in the individual with regard to causation and curtailment if not cure, their epistemological and clinical gaze should concentrate on faults in society. These societal faults include poverty, oppression and prejudice (Sheid and Brown, 2011), and as discussed above, a culture saturated with selfishness.

For Laing (1960) the main defect in Western society which affects the psyche is the configuration and operation of the nuclear family which he argues has led to interpersonal communicative strife between parents and their children. But, rather than this strife furnishing symptoms of insanity it produces signs of sanity. The affected person is acting rationally to a situation of irrationality. Laing's interest is in what conventional psychiatry devises as schizophrenia. But by extension his idea could cover, for example, depression, anxiety, manic-depression and narcissistic personality disorder. These supposed medical ailments of the mind/brain can be configured to be strategies for psychological survival.

Psychoanalyst, sociologist and philosopher Erich Fromm (1900–1980) takes the notion of rational response to societal fault to its logical conclusion. He postulates that virtually the entire population of the Western world is insane because Western society is itself insane. That is, there are not just aspects of society which cause madness but society is completely mad and this causes mass madness. An unanswered question is why Laing (who personally experienced familial discordant messages) and Fromm (who lived through two World Wars) should have been singularly sane enough to be able to observe and report the madness affecting others?

Fromm's 1955 book titled *The Sane Society* has sold millions of copies throughout the world (Friedman, 2013). It is in this book that he criticises the direction the Western world has taken and offers a blueprint for a better society. He points out that psychological adjustment to this insane society was not, as Laing would have it, reasonable human performance given the circumstances, but rather that it was ultimately detrimental to both the individual and human civilisation. Accepting society's crazy values and means of achieving these values is for Fromm not in any sense sensible. Moreover, what he refers to as the 'pathology of conformity' impelled by the powerful to pacify the general population, and by psychiatrists to tame their patients so that they could be rehabilitated into this passive population, does not reflect mental wellbeing but irrationality, ignorance and isolation.

People in the West, for Fromm (but apparently not Fromm) have become automatons, docilely submitting to and thereby reinforcing the social systems that contrive their crazy world and their own crazy way of being. Most people are not aware, and make little or no effort to become aware, that they are not being human or rather what Fromm has decided should be human. Humans in Western society have, for Fromm, become alienated from their 'self' due specifically to the capitalist mode of economic production which inspires a culture whereby humans perform un-humanly.

Intellectual inspiration

Fromm takes his intellectual inspiration from Karl Marx alongside Freud. Marx, in his masterpiece of economic theorising *Das Kapital* (1867; 1885; 1894), had pointed to the madness of the capitalist system. To continue to survive, capitalism requires increasingly sophisticated, means of finding and exploiting market opportunities otherwise the whole economic system would collapse. The collapse of capitalism for Marx as well as being desirable was inevitable. It was inevitable because, amongst other contradictions, capitalism's search for new markets contradicts the reality of the limit to expansion. So far, capitalism has survived by spreading rapidly across the globe, and in the process supplanting traditional cultural principles and practices that are otherwise alien to this form of economic production and its associated canons and customs. In its established centres of Europe, North America and Australasia, it has survived by fostering rampant consumerism, and commodity fetishism. Anything and everything is susceptible to capitalism's voracious and desperate appetite for new market opportunities. From this viewpoint, in the emerged economies of industrialised countries (based on manufacturing) and post-industrialised countries (characterised by service and finance), plus the emerging industrialising economies of countries such as China, Brazil, Russia, India and South Africa, material accumulation, and egocentrism have replaced or are replacing sharing and self-sacrifice, and unacknowledged generosity of spirit has been or will be superseded by the celebration of narcissism.

Marx had observed that at the offset, capitalism was capable of overlaying human needs with wants. That is, in its immature state it required workers to work so that they could and would aspire to buy products and to cultivate habits requiring further products which the workers had produced. The capitalists reaped the benefit of the monetary surplus by paying workers the difference between the cost of manufacturing the products, including the cost of labour, and the retail price. People then have to be prodded to buy these products, most of which are innovations, or renovations of previous necessities, rather than mere replacements for what have seemingly served as adequate up until that point. The prodding is especially effective when the fresh and freshened products are peddled and perceived as necessities.

The conversion of wants into needs is abetted by both advertising and the manipulation of supply and demand. For example, if public transport is starved of investment then more private cars can be sold as a 'needed' form of conveyance. However, Marx recognised that there is further manipulation regarding the choice made to satisfy capitalism's concocted needs. He realised that as capitalism proceeded, it was becoming extremely adept in selling consumers the all-encompassing message that 'we are what we buy' and that this is a natural way of life for humans. This idea has been taken up enthusiastically by theorists who are otherwise unenthusiastic about Marx's ideas, conspicuously his analysis of the social structure in past and present societies being broadly split into 'the haves' and the 'have nots', and his prediction that eventually communism would be the final and most equal society in which what everyone would have would be according to his/her needs. One grouping of critics, the postmodernists, whilst recognising that there is an 'underclass' which is left out of the main social system (due to, for example, severe economic or educational privation) proposes that most people living in contemporary capitalist economies are buying into having their wants satisfied as they already have their needs fulfilled.

Postmodern consumerism

Jean Baudrillard, who became a leading postmodernist theorist, was influenced by Marx particularly early in his academic career. One of his first books (he wrote dozens) is titled *La Société de Consommation* – translated as 'The Consumer Society' (Baudrillard, 1970). Here he suggests that the culture of consuming vast amounts of commodities is engaged in by people in Western countries as a way of making life meaningful. Meaningfulness from buying commodities becomes possible because of what he described as their 'sign-value'. Sign-value implies that commodities have significance beyond their practical worth. Moreover, different commodities have different sign-values, as do different commodities within a particular genre.

A tin of baked beans, money, bread, walking, breakfast cereals, houses, guns, sunglasses, clothing, death, teeth, wine, water, love, travelling and sex, have all been fetishised. That is, their sign-value is very much higher than their original use value. Take baked beans and sex. A tin of baked beans is no longer just a vessel containing a simple food nor sex sheer procreation. Beans and sex are inculcated with additional worth supplemental to, or as a replacement for, their original utility. The choice made about beans or sex revolves around their elemental purpose (sustenance and breeding), accepting that both, by-and-large, also have added pleasurable value if perhaps not to the same extent, *and* issues concerning the chooser's lifestyle.

A tenet of postmodern theorising is that there is in mature capitalist economies the freedom to make choices about lifestyle. However, having a choice is not straightforward. With regard to beans, what type should be bought from perhaps 57 varieties? Should it be a small tin, a large tin or a multipack, a supermarket own brand (speciously sometimes labelled as a 'value' product), and if so then from which supermarket should it be bought? Should it be a leading brand, and if so which leading brand? How much sugar and salt is acceptable, and what about the addition of sausages, bacon, or 'all-day-breakfast'? With regard to sex, which sort should be sought, from whom and from where? Which sexual identity should be adopted, heterosexual, homosexual, bisexual, metro-sexual or mono-sexual? Which sexual accoutrements might be included or protective measures taken? Asexuality may also be a choice out of disinterest, distaste or devoutness. Such freedom, as Laing observed (see Chapter 3), may have the deleterious psychological *sequelae* of ontological insecurity.

Material ownership ostensibly is pursued willingly and displayed freely in order to feel and project distinctiveness. For Baudrillard, however, the deeper and mostly unconscious reason for embracing consumerism is the attempt to avoid social isolation. No matter how nuanced the opportunities for differences are, within or between possessions or how active the consumer is in the acquisition, the desire to possess is a mass activity. Styles and fashions may come and go, but as they do there is a conjoint wave of humanity rejecting, demanding or grasping what has been, is or could be on offer. In such a world, reflects Baudrillard, alienation is complete as consumers are themselves consumed by a collective simulated existence in which needs and wants are indistinguishable. Separating needing from wanting is no longer feasible or required, and the need/want to obtain many former luxurious or superfluous commodities has become an expectation if not a right.

People in postmodern society (or what Marxists tend to refer to as late-modernity) according to Baudrillard exist in simulacra. That is, a substitute, or what he refers to as 'hyperreal', domain in which signs have replaced the real world (accepting that postmodernists tend to deny that there is any one authentic reality – or truth). The Internet, mobile phones, advertising, the media, and the excessive accumulation of possessions, provide a fantasy world in which people have swapped regular face-to-face connection for electronic means of association, and 'having' for humanness. They have themselves become objects.

Frankfurt School

Fromm's raised consciousness about how the economy of the Western world is responsible for pervasive and embedded derangement arose from a particular strand of Marxism. This strand was founded in the 1920s and became known the Frankfurt School of Critical Theory (Wolin, 2006; Wiggershaus, 2010). As is to be expected from those with an allegiance to Marxism, critical theorists are vehemently disapproving of capitalism. Less predictably they condemn the form of socialism dominated by the needs of the State, aided periodically by tyrannical leaders, characteristic of the now-defunct Union of Soviet Socialist Republics. They propose that an alternative path to human and social development is possible which can leave behind the repression of State-socialism and the inequities of capitalism.

Critical theory is 'critical' of capitalism and State-socialism because these systems foster an ideology which deliberately camouflages repression and inequality thereby furnishing a 'false consciousness' in their inhabitants about what is natural, actualising, and, emancipating. That there is this mystification of reality means people do not perform naturally as humans or reach their full potential. Fascism generates similar mystification largely out of fear.

For critical theorists the best method for understanding how these enchaining capitalist, State-socialist, and fascist systems work is through the intellectual process of critique aimed at digging below the surface of the relevant ideology which otherwise is presented as legitimate. Under (mature) capitalism people are indoctrinated by corporate business and their political allies into believing that individual needs and the insatiable consumption of commodities is normality. Under USSR-style State-socialism, it was the politburo and its bureaucracies which sold the 'collective' as having priority. Under fascism, it is the 'great leader' who formulates what is fitting for the nation whether this is infrastructure renewal or genocide. In each system, therefore, it is not just what people do but how they feel and think which is controlled. The Marxist Antonio Gramsci (1971) whilst imprisoned by the Italian Fascists in the 1920s used the term 'hegemony' in what became known as his 'prison notebooks' to describe how one group in society manages to convince the rest of the population of its political, economic, moral and legal authenticity to the point that it becomes accepted wisdom.

What the critical theorists attempt is to expose, through rigorous debate, how these societies actually operate. Such debating rigour, it is suggested, will reveal the hegemonic techniques which make the mass of people consent to subjugation. These self-appointed illuminators of truth combine intellectualism with activism. They seek to disseminate the inferences of their insights about how freedom is limited or non-existent for all but those with power. Thereby they hope to replace their targeted social system (or prevent, for example, the gestation of another State-socialist of fascist regime) into one which is emancipatory.

Alienated work

The main target for critique and change for Fromm was capitalism. Specifically, the themes of alienation, freedom, and the objectification of humanity are taken up by Fromm as the main elements of societal insanity under capitalism. For Fromm, capitalism and psychiatry have homogenised humanity and replaced human passions, spontaneity and intimacy with shopping and medication to mellow the spirits.

What Fromm advocates is the installing of a form of economic production which allows humans to reconnect with what they produce. Marx's point was that humans want to work creatively because this is an expression of their essential existence. A poignant example of the disconnection and the consequential estrangement of workers from their nature (at the time when Fromm was writing *The Sane Society*) was the assembly line. Workers on the assembly line simply had to be a cog in a machine. Often putting one cog into a machine was what they did all day and perhaps all their working lives. Each minute if not second of their working day would be monitored and regulated, with little time for interpersonal connection and no opportunity to play a part in the running of the factory. Such working conditions meant that their human creativity was ditched in favour of profitable production.

A poignant example from the twenty-first century, with similar dehumanising characteristics, is the multitude of battery-hen-like call centres employing millions globally. Call centre employees usually work from a script, have little or no expertise in their subject and are offered little or no opportunity to become expert. They are paid low wages, are supervised intensively, and are susceptible to emotional exhaustion due to frequent occurrences of hostile interactions with customers which can lead to withdrawal tactics as represented by high rates of absence (Deery *et al.*, 2002). A meta-analysis of research and theorising relating to alienation at work concludes, whilst acknowledging that employment conditions and employer–employee relations have become highly complex, that it continues to be a pertinent concept (Chiaburu *et al.*, 2014).

Capitalism's contradictions

Fromm's blueprint for a better society is revolutionary. He wants to iron-out the contractions which make the capitalist economy unreasonable (that is both irrational and iniquitous). However, more than merely making work meaningful once again, Fromm wants to make human life more meaningful generally by radically changing the whole of society. That is, .he wants to liberate humans from the inhuman shackle of hollow and exploitative employment *and* the puerile cultural outpourings of an economic system which lauds money and what it can buy – power and possessions. Fromm, therefore, follows the classic Marxist proposition that the economic base of a society is responsible for the shape and substance not only of work but of all aspects society. The ways in which its institutions function and the ways in which people behave, feel, and think, are directly and indirectly directed by the requirements of the economic system and this is so no matter what type of system.

The capitalist economic system, argues Fromm, has terrible social penalties for those who are contained by it and for those who threaten its continuation. Wars are fought in which millions die to defend trading markets. Economic trading cycles produce periods of high employment and then periods of high unemployment. Whichever part of the economic cycle capitalism is in vast differences are maintained between those who have power and possessions and those who are disempowered and dispossessed.

Adopting Fromm's Marxist-orientated perspective, far from a sane blueprint it can be argued that as the globalisation of Western-inspired capitalism has proliferated there is concomitant flourishing of social insanity. Western-inspired capitalism has become the dominant economic system and one which has concentrated power and possessions in an outstandingly privileged minority.

Data from three sources (Oxfam, 2014; Credit Suisse, 2015; World Bank, 2016) indicate that global wealth is expanding, the middle classes are growing, and there are increasing numbers of billionaires, but also that wealth inequality is widening vastly and there is a large poverty-stricken population:

- Half of the world's wealth is owned by just one per cent of the population and 10 per cent own nearly 88 per cent.
- Seven out of 10 people live in countries where economic inequality has increased in the last 30 years.
- The richest one per cent increased their share of income in 24 out of 26 countries between 1980 and 2012.
- In 2015 over 700 million people are living in dire poverty.

Wealth and poverty cannot be linked straightforwardly with power and disempowerment respectively. There are complex dynamics operating at the individual and societal levels with regard to where power lies (Lukes, 2004). However, wealth is a, if not the, most significant resource in exercising power in political arenas. Above and beyond factors such as educational attainment, inherited or achieved social status, entrepreneurial spirit, and military might (all of which may be connected to wealth either as precursors or corollaries), sizeable incomes and/or considerable assets are used to gain political power. Moreover, prosperous proprietors of large national and transnational corporations, whilst not a coherent and conscious group, are senior members of a global power elite (Mills, 1956; Domhoff, 2014). This elite or 'superclass' which contains the very wealthy, high-ranking politicians, military chiefs, media moguls and business leaders, stands above all other social classes. It is far more influential than the upper class and overrides the democratic process because power is frequently exercised covertly and stealthily rather than through the ballot box and parliamentary procedure.

During 2007/8 the international financial system neared collapse in part due to the impenetrable density of its organisations and systems. But it was also due to the irresponsibility, avarice and arrogance of a significant element of the superclass, the financiers, bankers, and regulators (Davies, 2010; Kay, 2015). They fit Twenge and Campbell's description of 'normal narcissists'. Ironically, and presumably unwittingly, these financial roguish self-seekers were participating in the perpetrating of what could have been the ultimate contradiction in capitalism – the one which would lead to its complete downfall. Threats of economic collapse remain (Pope Francis, 2014; International Monetary Fund, 2015).

Corporate psychopathy

Joel Bakan, Professor of Law at the University of British Columbia, Canada, points to other institutional and individual perpetrators of pecuniary conceit. In his book *The Corporation* (2004) and in the film of the same name, he presents the argument that corporations, mainly the larger ones, act psychopathically and are in the long run dysfunctional for society. If success is measured by profit then successful businesses benefit employees because of increased job security and wages being paid, shareholders benefit because there are elevated dividends, and governments benefit because more tax is attained. However, for Bakan, the pursuit of profit by big business is wrecking physical environments across the world, and wrecking the lives of millions of workers who may receive minimal reward for alienating employment and who may at the profit-motivated whim of a company's executive board be made unemployed. Moreover, the profit-making ethos of big business is largely responsible for the pandemic of materialism, commodification, consumerism and thus a culture of narcissism.

Bakan invited Robert Hare to contribute to *The Corporation* by assessing corporate psychopathy. A renowned criminal psychologist, author of *Without Conscience: The Disturbing World of the Psychopaths Among Us* (Hare, 1999), Hare is also the architect of what has become the standard tool for diagnosing psychopathy. Hare assessed a selection of business institutions and concluded that if these institutions were human they would be certified as psychopathic. Moreover, the concern shown by corporations over the damage done to the environment and to people when exposed by the media or campaign groups, and their instigation of programmes of social responsibility serve only to manipulate public and political opinion:

> Human psychopaths are notorious for their ability to use charm as a mask to hide their dangerously self-obsessed personalities. For corporations, social responsibility may play the same role.
>
> *Hare quoted in Bakan, 2004, p.56*

Using the corporate tactic of social responsibility corporations can present as compassionate and community-spirited. But, corporations, for Hare, are essentially selfish.

However, Hare maintains that the psychopathy of corporations does not necessarily arise from the performance of the individuals who make up their executive. Most executives have families and friendships which do appear to be imbued with genuineness. Some of the most successful business magnates contribute business sizeable proportions of their wealth to philanthropy. For example, Bill Gates (co-founder of Microsoft), along with his wife Melinda, and Warren Buffet (a hugely successful financial investor) have given billions of USA dollars to a charitable foundation which has the aim of reducing poverty and ill health in Africa (Gates Foundation, 2015). However, some executives says Hare, are psychopathic.

Hare and psychologist Paul Babiak, who specialises in corporate management and leadership, were to claim two years after Bakan's book was published that big business was infested with psychopaths (Babiak and Hare, 2006). This, they suggest, is because those with psychopathic tendencies have an advantage when seeking promotion to executive level in corporations. Those they refer to as the 'snakes in suits' are over-represented in executive positions compared with the incidence of psychopathy in the general population. Babiak and Hare comment that those who can charm their colleagues including their bosses, are risk-takers, and may well be very intelligent, articulate and objective. Eventually, however, they are dysfunctional for the businesses in which they are employed. Their valued corporate qualities become displaced by their exorbitant egotism.

Had Fromm been alive in the twenty-first century he also might have opined that the superclass has become exorbitantly insane because it seems to be presiding over the collapse of human life if not all life on planet Earth. Global warming is agreed to be happening by the vast majority of natural scientists (Cook *et al.*, 2013), the USA National Aeronautics and Space Administration (NASA, 2014), the International Panel of Climate Change (IPCC, 2015), the World Meteorological Organization (2016), and affirmed by a host of environmental campaigners (for example, Gore, 2006; Lovelock, 2010; Klein, 2015). It is also agreed that the cause of global warming is probably human activity stemming from past Western and present global outpourings of manufacturing and service industrialisation which feeds consumerism and commodification. The continued inability or disinclination of governments and corporations to install and abide by a measure of global governance aimed at averting the tipping point beyond which lies ecological calamity is not sane. Moreover, the superclass, by not pulling back from the tipping point (and not controlling its psychopathic sub-section), might well have been considered by Fromm as super-insane *and* super-stupid. The uncomfortable truth, however, is that whilst the global elite can be justifiably accused of being selfish monkeys, to use Liddle's phrase, so might be the global public.

That humanity *per se* is culpably imprudent is the position taken by Stephen Emmott. Emmott is head of Microsoft's Computational Science research, Visiting Professor of Biological Computation at University College London, and Visiting Professor of Computational Science at the University of Oxford. In his book *10 Billion* (Emmott, 2013), he argues that humanity is doomed because the public along with business and political leaders have failed to install fundamental changes to how the world's remaining natural resources are used which with a global population rising to 10 billion in the coming decades are unsustainable. For Emmott, the tipping point has been reached and is heading resolutely towards environmental disaster. Gloomily and fatalistically he predicts that there isn't anything that has yet been proposed (such as scientific inventiveness or profound conversion in human lifestyle which leaves behind materialism) nor anything likely to be proposed (and universal population control remains a taboo proposition) that humans and their leaders are likely to adopt which will reverse the tipping direction.

Dumbing down

The engrossment and exploitation of individuals in stupidity occurs also, contends Fromm, in the area of culture in the sense of everyday pursuits having become dumbed-down since the 1950s in the West. Western culture has succumbed to commodification promulgated purely for financial yield. Human intimacy, intellectual improvement, appreciation of the arts, is traded for superficial and unfulfilling mass entertainment. Just as meaningful work had become meaningless, high-brow recreation was becoming low-brow.

For Fromm, despite most of the population being literate and having access to such potentially mind-expanding technologies of radio, television and film, as well as newspapers, what is actually provided and sought is uneducated, ill-informed, mind-narrowing, cultural garbage:

> [I]nstead of giving us the best of the past and present literature and music, these media of communication, supplanted by advertising, fill the minds of men with the cheapest of trash, lacking in any sense of reality, with sadistic phantasies.
>
> *Fromm, 1955, p.5*

Had Fromm seen out a century of life he probably would have been startled at how low-brow and widespread such cultural garbage had become. A few examples of what might have stupefied a centenarian Fromm about how far human stupidity had come include: the prevalence and triteness of electronic social media; 'reality' television programmes which concentrate on the humiliation of participants from the public; the daily diet of shallow commentary, malicious gossip and sensationalism in popular newspapers and magazines; the commonness of carnage and cruelty in films; the corporate takeover of sport; the demeaning and commercialisation of sexuality through the spread of pornography (largely on the Internet); bingeing on alcohol; the rise of religious and political fundamentalism; the notion of 'creative design'; the seemingly insatiable appetite for shopping (Mosely, 2000; Measham and Brain, 2005; Bauerlein, 2008; Carr, 2011; Dimofte *et al.*, 2015).

But what could demonstrate the continuing folly of humanity more than the continuation of lethal encounters and the consequential disruption or destruction of States and mass movements of people. Over the last 2,000 years, the trend in violence by humans against other humans has been downwards (Pinker, 2012). Nevertheless, both fatal and non-fatal violence remain a major social and health problem globally (United Nations Office on Drugs and Crime; 2014; World Health Organisation, 2014b). In recent decades civil wars, failing and failed states and terrorism, has resulted in more than 10 million deaths, and hundreds of millions of refugees and migrants (Hanhimäki and Blumenau, 2013; Howard, 2014; United Nations Population Fund, 2015; United Nations, 2016).

Individualism and collectivism

What Fromm wanted politically was 'humanistic communitarian socialism' which he believed would be exemplified by creative work, loving relationships, comradeship, compromise, as well as individuality. Fromm's backing of individuality is congruent with his psychoanalytic background. Psychoanalysis, as with all psychotherapy, concentrates on the 'psyche' not on society. It is the person, not his/his culture or community laying down or sitting next to the therapist (Morrall, 2008). The humanistic part of Fromm's political bent, which implies individuals and their aspirations are paramount, does seem to clash with communitarianism and socialism both of which imply commitment to the collective. However, Fromm argued consistently for personal and political freedom, and for individuals to take responsibility for both. He proposes that for humans to be fully free (and sane) they have to escape the tyranny of their own fears about what they can achieve for themselves. They also have to escape from the tyranny of political regimes which pursue social injustice and prevent individual accomplishment.

Freud did have a sociological bent which led him to appreciate the important effect of society on the individual, for example, in the socialisation of the superego (that is the individual's conscience). Indeed, Freud is considered as a key thinker in psychology *and* sociology (Bocock, 2002). Equally, Fromm brings together psychology and sociology by recognising the cultural causative elements in the development of selfishness and narcissism. Selfishness and narcissism were for Fromm paradoxical symptoms. He suggested that what furnishes selfishness is not the individual's fondness for him/herself but a lack of fondness for him/herself. This lack of fondness endows constant anxiety in that person about who and what they really are. The narcissistic person has similar internal contradictions. Whilst he/she seems on the surface to be enthralled by his/her personage this is compensation for deep self-loathing (Fromm, 1939).

With selfishness and narcissism, Fromm brings together dynamics of the psyche with cultural patterns, personality traits and social pressures which connect to formulate instrumental but not genuine self-love. Capitalist society requires the self-centred consumption of commodities but not intellectual, emotional and behavioural self-actualisation. Humans reaching for the pinnacle of their potential performance would not be functional to a materialistic social system.

The trouble with Fromm's various answers for replacing an alienating, dehumanising society which arouses selfishness, and narcissism is that they are imprecise, romanticised and condescending. He does offer some precise exemplars (such as communes and workers-cooperatives) and stratagems (for example, a combination of World Government and localised 'town hall' politics, and education for self-improvement and for life). Moreover, he argues that the ideal moral, philosophical and spiritual precepts for a better society are already known. They can be found in the Judeo-Christian teachings (Islam is not mentioned) and humanism, although as an atheist God would not figure in Fromm's brave new world of 'collective art', singing, dancing, sculpting, painting and self and communal love. However, a detailed and credible plan for a revolutionary reconfiguration of insane capitalism into sane humanistic communitarian socialism is missing. Crucially, he does not pinpoint practical and ideological mechanisms for undoing the hegemonic moulding of the masses which has turned them into mad materialists.

Moreover, the assertion that there is a 'worse' society from which people need to be freed and a 'better' society in which people will be free is a God-like commandment from the non-God believing Fromm. Put bluntly, who or what gives Fromm (or any individual) the right or insight to decide how a 'freed humanity' should live? Collective artistry, singing and dancing are not for everyone.

Continuing insanity

Fromm's recommendations for social change, no matter how prescriptive, have not been administered. Since *The Sane Society* was published there has been more commodification and consumerism, an increase in inequality and further concentration of power, a population explosion in the selfish-monkey troop, and an escalation of low-brow culture. Society has become more rather than less insane.

That said, it has become *de rigour* in social science and psychiatry to acknowledge that madness has social connotations. The World Health Organisation readily accepts that factors external to the individual biological and psychological make-up, especially inequality, affect the condition of a person's mind:

> A person's mental health and many common mental disorders are shaped by various social, economic, and physical environments operating at different stages of life. Risk factors for many common mental disorders are heavily associated with social inequalities, whereby the greater the inequality the higher the inequality in risk.
>
> *World Health Organisation/Gulbenkian Foundation, 2014, p.9*

Although poverty inexorably exacerbates susceptibility to and the experience of madness, it is inequality which is identified repeatedly by researchers and health organisations as a major factor in furnishing madness in societies which are not poverty-stricken (Friedi, 2009; Wilkinson and Pickett, 2010; Mental Health Foundation, 2013).

The idea that society itself is mad by tolerating inequality and encouraging patterns of human performance geared to fetishising commodities, indulgence in mindless mass media, celebrity and narcissism, at the expense of intimacy, communality and aesthetic and intellectual pursuits, is not generally accepted. However, such a position has been reiterated by a few social thinkers since Fromm first proposed such a radical analysis. One of these is psychologist Oliver James (2007; 2008). James attacks 'selfish capitalism' in the West and presently spreading globally, for upholding an ideology which cherishes rampant materialism. This excessive materialism, he argues, has created a social infection he terms 'affluenza'. When infected by affluenza people live their lives striving to get meaning from buying, accumulating and displaying products. James suggests that selfish capitalism should be replaced by unselfish capitalism whereas Fromm prescribes replacing capitalism (and totalitarianism) to cure the insanity of society.

A practitioner of integrative medicine, Frank Lipman (2009) argues that the materialism of contemporary capitalism has pushed the pace of living to the point whereby many people have become 'spent'. That is, the Internet, mobile phones, multiple television channels, long hours commuting to work and then long hours and longer years working, continuously trying to increase earnings whilst increasing indebtedness, residing and seeking recreation in jam-packed cities, and jamming-in holidays using heaving transport systems, eating high-calorie foods and having the opportunity to shop perpetually either on-line or in 24-hour high-street retail outlets, having multiple choices to make over similar products, a deluge of advertisements reaching into our homes and spread throughout public spaces, all contribute to physical and psychological collapse. This busyness, Lipman argues, has been activated by the profit needs of business not the natural needs of humans. Journalist Madeleine Bunting posits that we have become 'willing slaves' to the corporate model whereby nothing is enough and even everything would not satisfy. Yet here is another contradiction of the capitalist economic system. Just as an actualised self is not really functional to capitalism neither is a spent slave.

Fry in the Bunting sense can be regarded as mindfully submissive to the incessant demands of corporate media. But such demands, Fry infers, have led him close to irrevocable dysfunction:

> Stephen Fry has said that he finds his celebrity 'exhausting' and that there's every possibility he'd consider suicide one day.
>
> *PinkNews, 2011*

Fry was to confess that he had attempted suicide the following year by taking a mixture of drugs and alcohol (BBC News, 2013). The year after Fry was to tour the UK to promote his latest autobiographical text, *More Fool Me*, he had been voted the 'most loved' celebrity (again) on the social media site Twitter (Griffiths, 2014). He presented a talk on 'Shakespeare and Love' at the respected British Hay Festival of Literature and Arts, and continued to appear regularly on television and radio, to name but a few of his exhausting celebrity events. In 2016, Fry disclosed yet more detail about his self-imposed gruelling lifestyle and efforts at self-destruction in the fittingly titled follow-up to his previous documentary, *The Not So Secret Life of the Manic Depressive: 10 Years On*.

Fromm's contradictions

Furthermore, there is a fundamental aberration in Fromm's thinking. He highlights the increased incidence of mental disorder as an indicator of capitalism's contrariness. As capitalism becomes more embedded and successful if measured by economic growth there is an exponential embedding and growth in social stress and psychological distress, with up to a quarter of the population of countries such Britain and the USA diagnosed with a mental disorder (Wilkinson and Pickett, 2010). However, it is not logical for Fromm to use the increased rate of mental disorder as an indication of the insanity of society. His primary position is that society is insane and that makes all or most of its occupants insane. If this is so, then mental disorder must be an aberrant social phenomenon. Alternatively, mental disorder could be a magnified state of normal madness. What it cannot be if Fromm is to be consistent, is a sign of generalised insanity as that would mean that now or eventually everyone would have a diagnosis of, for example, personality disorder, schizophrenia or manic-depression. No matter how extensive the reach of the DSM, it is yet to go beyond medicalising a minority.

Moreover, Fromm's assessment of capitalism attends to its contradictions but fails to mention its contribution to the betterment of humankind. Social advancements in fully-fledged capitalist countries embrace longer lifespans, less infant and maternal mortality, and a plethora of technological discoveries and effective medical interventions.

Cecil Helman

Western psychiatry, as has been deliberated above, tends to ignore or underplay the role of society in the origin and formation of madness. This has been a long-standing inclination (Eisenberg and Kleinman, 1980; Kaplan et al., 1996; James in Wessely and James, 2013).

Societal sources and/or signifiers of insanity have been, however, recognised by psychiatry in one very particular and peculiar way as far back as the days of its founders such as Esquirol (Cox, 1986). The past convention in psychiatry has been to refer to a group of disorders as 'culture-bound'. These culture-bound disorders were construed as confined mainly to non-Western areas of the world. This recognition has been underscored by the willingness of some medical practitioners to engage with anthropology. Cross-cultural or trans-cultural psychiatry today includes attention to clinical issues of culture not only between but within societies (Leseth, 2015).

Society and culture

Cecil Helman (1944–2009) was a family physician and distinguished medical anthropologist, and author of the standard textbook on how culture affects health (titled *Culture, Health and Illness*). This was first published in 1984 and has run to five editions. Anthropology is the study of humans in the context of their culture. Culture is more difficult to define and to separate from a definition of society. Society for sociologist Lord Antony Giddens (2009) is expressed as the particular political, economic, legal and civil institutions and associated organisational processes and systems of a geographically bounded group. Culture for Giddens is described as the accepted and shared customs, values and moral codes, of a socially coherent group. Helman (2007) conflates these two definitions as I tend to do because of the 'multicultural' characteristic of many societies. The multifarious patterns of migration, the rise of effects of global capitalism and cyber-society make a distinction between society and culture unfeasible if not irrelevant.

Medical anthropology for Helman it is the study of human health and illness in the relevant cultural context. Helman provides more detail:

> [Medical anthropology] is about how people in different cultures and social groups explain the causes of ill health, the types of treatment they believe in, and to whom they turn if they do get ill … [and] how these beliefs and practices relate to biological, psychological and social changes in the human organism.
>
> *Helman, 2007, p.2*

Hence for Helman, medical practitioners, whether dealing with physical or mental disorder, cannot comprehend properly health and disease, and the patient's suffering, unless his/her cultural context, including attitudes to life, death, pain and happiness, is appreciated and treatment is adjusted accordingly which may mean not offering any medical intervention.

Relativity and universality

Helman's medical anthropological approach intimates a major and possibly insurmountable quandary faced by anthropologists and psychiatrists alike in trying to understanding madness. Can madness be categorised as universal or relative to a culture? Hearing voices or seeing visions, believing in homeopathy or celebrity, or acting with maniacal certitude or melancholic insecurity, may on the one hand be indicative of madness or normality depending on the culture in which they are aired. On the other hand some human performances (for example, cannibalism) may be attributed to insanity and/or criminality in a society, many societies or globally, no matter what the cultural features. It is axiomatic that this dilemma applies to many, perhaps all, aspects of human performance. The question then broadens to become: are most if not all normal and abnormal kinds of thinking, feeling and behaving, 'culture-bound' or 'culturally-unbound'?

Helman records that apparent conditions of culture, such as spirit possession (and witchcraft), appear in many parts of the world and at many different historical points including the twenty-first century and are not attendant on a state of madness. But, he argues, this does not mean that spirit possession can be viewed as normal even within those areas and epochs. The majority of people in those places where, and at those times when spirit possession does transpire will never themselves be overcome by spirits monstrous or not. Moreover, instances of spirit possession are irregular. He suggests that the appearance (in both senses of the word) of possession relies on a set of cultural values and practices, especially those connected to religion, which allow interpersonal and social strife to be framed in this way. Without these there could be no substance for the specific spirit form of possession or any concept of spirit possession in the first place:

> Possession then, is an 'abnormal' form of individual behaviour, but one that conforms with cultural values, and whose expression is closely controlled by cultural norms.
>
> *Helman, 2007, p.248*

These norms, posits Helman, frame the circumstances and content of the possession, and the ways in which it can be recognised and dealt with by others.

Penis-retraction and sexual-hysteria

Helman is hitting the middle-ground *within* the medical model of madness between 'culture-bound' and 'culturally-unbound' madness. Anthropology is much more consenting to the social constructionist perspective with its intermittent forays into the farthest reaches of relativism whereby no one culture takes epistemological, moral, normative, legal, or indeed medical, precedence over another unless by force, indoctrination or acquiescence. The knowledge, beliefs and practices of each culture are taken as legitimate by and only for that culture, and cannot be transferred to other cultures. Psychiatry's approach to the validity of the cultural content of predicaments of the mind has been erratic and remains unsettled but has overall been moving in the direction of universality (Cooper, 2010).

At one end of this meandering medicalised terrain in which Helman places himself half-way, is a small stack of mental disorders which only appear in certain cultural settings but are or were considered as authentic disorders by psychiatry, and which are also usually considered abnormal by the population in whose culture they occur. The notion that there are these 'culture-bound' mental disorders has long been chronicled by psychiatry as well as anthropology (Hirst and Woolley, 1982; Cox, 1986). Examples include 'Koro' which is a disorder originally thought to happen to Chinese men but has also been recorded in Nigeria, Singapore, Thailand and India. The (male) Koro sufferer experiences an episode of panic because he believes his penis is retracting into his abdomen. This is worrying enough but his overriding fear is that should his abdomen manage to seize said penis then death will ensue. Arctic Inuit females more often than men are susceptible to the disorder of 'Pibloktoq'. Outbursts of crying, speaking in tongues (glossolalia), and manic episodes involving frantic running, frequently naked, over the ice-bound terrain and possibly into icy water, followed by deep-sleep events (presumably if not frozen to death in the meantime), and amnesia on waking about the foregone events.

At the other end of the terrain in which Helman sits equidistant is a vast stack of mental disorders which can appear in any cultural setting, and increasingly are considered as universally abnormal and medically authentic by psychiatry (Cooper, 2010). Koro has been deemed an anxiety-state brought on by feelings of guilt over sexual indiscretion, and Pibloktoq as hysteria generated by gender and sexual subordination (although ironically hysteria is no longer unequivocally accepted by psychiatry as a precise disorder).

Arthur Kleinman

Arthur Kleinman (1941–) is Professor of Medical Anthropology and Professor of Psychiatry at Harvard University. In 1986 he founded the journal *Culture, Medicine and Psychiatry*. As has Helman, he pioneered the comprehension and application of anthropological ideas in medical practice, but his focus has been on doing so in psychiatry.

Category fallacy

Kleinman uses the concept of 'category fallacy' to criticise the imperialistic tendencies of psychiatrists:

> The category fallacy ... The reification of one culture's diagnostic categories and their projection onto patients in another culture, where those categories lack coherence and their validity has not been established, is a category fallacy.
>
> *Kleinman, 1988, p.15*

Kleinman does not dismiss altogether the legitimacy of some psychiatric categories such as schizophrenia which for him may have universal application. However, he does rail against the presumption of supremacy by psychiatry. Using an argument which may seem similar to that propounded by Szsaz (see Chapter 3), he suggests that many if not most of the 'culture-bound' disorders along with Western-based disorders may be labelled medical sometimes and in some places but could become labelled as, for example, moral, criminal or religious problems on other occasions.

The similarity with Szasz is perfunctory, however, as he recoils from the idea that most mental disorders are not real. He declares his allegiance to his (medical) profession and his disgust at the anti-psychiatry movement (remembering Szsaz does not regard himself as an anti-psychiatrist) for, in all likelihood unwittingly, not taking the suffering of the mentally disordered seriously. Kleinman's view is similar to that of Helman in that he wants more 'culture' to be embedded in psychiatric practice.

Helman's compromise position is to accept the legitimacy of mental disorder, but that legitimacy must depend on the inclusion in the clinical setting of the 'collective viewpoint' arising from patients' and clinicians' respective cultures. That is for Helman the medical practitioner in primary care and specialist services for the mentally disordered must be alert to the cultural contexts which affect both causes and effect with regard to mental disorder otherwise diagnoses and treatments will almost certainly be misinformed and misdirected.

Most anthropologists have tended towards the relativist position (Hatch, 1983). Most psychiatrists have inclined towards universalism (Featherstone, 2005). Contemporary psychiatry, however, does espouse a degree of Helman-type cultural sensitivity in its defining, listing and treatment of mental disorders. The DSM-V (American Psychiatric Association, 2013) makes reference to all forms of psychological distress as being shaped by culture including the hundreds of disorders listed in that manual. However, it has reduced its list of 25 culture-bound syndromes in its previous edition to nine of what are described as 'the best-studied concepts' of psychological distress from around the world. The shortened list includes *ataque de nervios* (an attack of 'nerves' – Hispanic communities), *khyâl cap* (a 'wind' attack – Cambodian refugees), and *Kufungisisa* (an attack of thinking – Zimbabwe). Windigo Psychosis does not make an appearance in the DSM-V, or in the revised 2010 World Health Organisation's International Classification of Disease (ICD-10).

The apparent sensitising of psychiatry to culture, however, has furthered insensitivity to lucidity. The category of 'culture-bound syndromes' in the DSM-V has been superseded by three concepts: (a) cultural syndromes: clusters of symptoms which tend occur amongst individuals in specific cultural groups, communities; (b) cultural idioms of distress: expressions of distress that may not involve specific symptoms; (c) cultural explanations of distress: local understandings of cause and effect concerning psychological distress. It is difficult to see how a clinician, particularly a generalist medical practitioner, could be expected to unpack these concepts besides the need to unpick syndromes contained a cultural hue from the hundreds not contaminated by culture. Moreover, the whole notion of context of any sort interfering with a diagnosis of mental disorder or normality has been questioned by Professor of Psychiatry, Roland Pies:

> Context does not dissolve disorder, even if it seems to explain it. And often, we are quite wrong about such seeming explanations.
>
> *Pies, 2013, p.1*

The World Psychiatric Association transcultural-psychiatry section, whose membership is open to psychologists and anthropologists, sets out principles and objectives directed towards exploring similarities and differences across and between cultures in how mental disorder is caused, how it presents, and which treatments are the most appropriate based on 'evidence' and 'values', Its values, however, may be judged skewed towards Western culture and psychiatric dominance given that two of its principles refer to fostering psychiatry for all people of the world and the protection of the rights of psychiatrists (World Psychiatric Association, 2015a).

Swift runner

The story of Swift Runner (real name Ka-Ki-Si-Kutchin) lays bare the confounding character of cultural variance and interrelated problematics of erroneous classifications, psychiatric imperialism and relativism versus universality. Swift Runner was a First Nation Algonquian-Cree who lived in nineteenth century British colonial Canada. He was a hunter and trapper and sometime guide for the North Western Mounted Police (the 'Mounties'). In 1879 Swift Runner was legally executed at Fort Saskatchewan, Alberta. He had been found guilty of cannibalism having eaten his wife, children, and one or two other relatives (Thomson, 1984; Library and Archives Canada, 1994).

Every narrative about every person or event can begin at any point at the arbitrary discretion of the narrator. I (arbitrarily) start the story of Swift Runner as he returns alone from what was to be later adjudicated as the scene of his crimes.[1] He is seeking shelter in the Catholic Mission in St. Albert and this is given to him by the priests who presumably knew him and his family. This is in the spring of 1879. The previous winter, which seemingly was exceptionally harsh, he and his family had been camping in woods to the north-east of Edmonton. Swift Runner is fortunate to have been given shelter at the Mission, but this kindness is to prove his nemesis.

The priests at the Mission are not convinced by his explanation for the absence of his wife, children and other relatives. His explanation is that they have all starved to death due to the extreme weather resulting in them not being able to hunt or forage for food. The problem that the priests have with this account is that first he is alive and second he is not malnourished. This begged the questions: why had he been the only one to survive? Why has he survived so well? Their suspicion is aroused further because during his stay in the Mission he has regular screaming fits whilst sleeping. The priests ask for an explanation from him for these nocturnal disturbances. He attributes his outbursts to being possessed by a spirit. Claims of spirit possession in traditional cultures across Africa, Asia, and in Japan, are well-known and well documented (Laycock, 2014). What the possessed believe is that their minds and bodies have been taken over by an external force. This external force may be an ancestor, a divinity, a ghost or ogre. Those people claiming to be possessed by a spirit are frequently believed by their communities (Boddy, 1994)

The priests are not likely to have been surprised by his account of possession given that they were living in close proximity to people from such tribes as the Cree and did believe what he said as truthful. What Swift Runner tells his clerical inquisitors is that it is the 'Windigo Monster' which has possessed him.

The Windigo Monster was believed by Algonquian Indians to incite those it possessed with cannibalistic urges (Carlson, 2009). This the priests know. The priests, therefore, report what Swift Runner has told them to the police, the North West Mounted force (the 'Mounties') with whom Swift Runner had worked previously as a guide. He is escorted by the police to where he and his family had camped for the winter. Here the police find human remains. Eventually, he tells one of the priests, Father Hippolyte Leduc, what he says is 'the truth' and his statement is used in his prosecution.

> First I shot my son the next to the eldest, the eldest one [I] stoned to death, I shot my second boy ... I shot my wife through the breast, the two little girls I knocked in the head with an axe, I choked the baby girl ... my eldest boy died of starvation.
> Signed: Ka-Ki-Si-Kutchin
>
> *Library and Archives Canada, 1997*

Although, the number of deaths for which he was culpable alters depending on whether Swift Runner's confession, official documents or newspapers, is the source, it would seem he had murdered and eaten up to nine members of his family.

The trial took place on 6 August 1879 at Fort Saskatchewan in the province of Alberta with Judge High Richardson presiding. The court documents refer to Swift Runner being above average intelligence of 'any Indian' and him not showing 'any apparent symptom of insanity'. When asked if he had any witnesses to call or anything to say in his defence to the jury he is reported to have replied 'No. I did it'. He was duly found guilty not of mass murder and/or cannibalism but of murdering one family member, his wife. The death sentence was passed. A recommendation for mercy was either not made or if made not given. On 20 of December 1879 Swift Runner was hanged.

That Swift Runner was executed implies that he was viewed by the legal authorities as bad not mad. His confession underscores a malevolent but rational reason for his killing spree – he slaughtered and ingested his family to save himself from starvation, and in additional statements to Father Hippolyte Leduc he admits as much. The court is told that he is bright 'for any Indian' and is not suffering from mental disorder. That he may have been possessed by the spirit of the Windigo Monster appears not to have mattered much to him given that he did not use it as a defence, nor did it matter to the court given that he was sentenced to death.

So what is it that psychiatrists have had to say about Swift Runner and the Windigo Monster? They have said a lot but much of what has been said from this quarter is incongruous to the original trial decision and contradictory over time. Moreover, initial thinking from anthropologists over the status of Swift Runner's mind and the Windigo Monster contributed to the psychiatric position(s) and to the confusion.

The contribution from a Reverend John Cooper (1933), a Catholic anthropologist, typifies the thinking of both psychiatry and anthropology for many years about what became classified as a severe and dangerous mental disorder, Windigo Psychosis. Cooper claimed that this condition was common amongst the Cree and other tribes living in close proximity. It is, he suggests, characterised by an unnatural craving to eat human flesh. He also refers to how the Windigo has a heart of ice, some of which it may decide to vomit. For Cooper, the account of the Windigo is born out of Cree folklore but that does not make it mythical. The spirit possession is experienced as real as is the ensuing madness. Moreover, Cooper blames what he calls the 'prevalent cultural conditions' (p.24) of the Cree lifestyle for the presence of the Monster which possesses Swift Runner. Reverend Emile Saindon, another Catholic anthropologist and an associate of Cooper, supplies particulars about these cultural conditions affecting the James Bay Cree. He also provides his thoughts on contributing biological elements, psychological traits, and features of the physical environment causing what he describes as 'Indian Fear' of which he claims 'Windigo sickness' is a sub-set:

> [D]efective physical hygiene, malnutrition, menstrual disorders, tuberculosis, overindulgence in tea-drinking, inclement climate and hard environment, pathological heredity, the unmasking of recessive defects through close inbreeding, and last but not least, faulty training and lack of firm discipline.
>
> *Saindon, 1933, pp.1–2*

Whilst the inclusion of faulty individual and societal factors is insightful with regard to what might instigate a possessed mind, the manner and substance of Saindon's list of factors provides insight into the colonial mind. Both Reverends were writing for a Catholic anthropological journal with the title 'Primitive Man'. What perhaps is primitive is the way in which data were collected and opinions affirmed by the early anthropologists, which in turn was to influence psychiatrists.

Psychiatry's cultural arm aided and abetted by anthropology, had for many decades during the nineteenth century and into the twentieth century assumed that the Cree and other Algonquian tribes believed in the Windigo, assumed that spirit possession did actually happen as far as these tribes were concerned, assumed that possession by the Windigo could lead and did lead in some cases to cannibalism, and assumed that this particular form of possession was a 'culture-bound' mental disorder.

Anthropologists' dilemma

The latter assumption gives rises to an investigative and epistemological quandary which is related to the relativity–universality debate. This is the perennial anthropologist's dilemma: if a culture is studied by a researcher (objectively) from another culture then the culture under study may not be understood properly because his/her observations will be moulded by the values and practices provided by the culture of origin; if the researcher becomes absorbed into the culture under study, or if an inhabitant of that culture is the researcher, in order to understand it properly (subjectively) then his/her observations will be moulded by the values and practices of the culture being studied (Hirst and Woolley, 1982). A resolution of the anthropologist's dilemma is fundamental to resolving which if any madness/mental disorders are culture-bound and which if any are culturally-unbound.

Mythical Monster

Arising from the anthropologist's dilemma being unresolved, as well as from large dollops of colonial prejudice and ignorance, the assumptions listed above about the Windigo all turned out to be misleading or just plain wrong. According to anthropologist Seymour Parker (1960), the Cree did not believe that the Windigo was anything more than a myth, a story made-up to frighten and control adolescents into undertaking certain coming-of-age practices. There was not a real ice-hearted monster ready and waiting to infuse its victims with cannibalistic cravings but only a pretend one invented by adults to persuade children to become adults. Cannibalism did occur amongst many traditional tribes in North America and elsewhere. The reasons for cannibalism in traditional tribal communities were varied, for example, indisputable food scarcity, totemic demonstration of tribal superiority (and was used by colonists for this purpose), or a funeral rite by which the soul of a dead loved-one could be incorporated into the body of the living, and feasting on the remains of human sacrifice to appease particular gods (Barker et al., 1998; Feldman, 2008). Parker observes that none of those anthropologists who in the 1930s espoused ideas about Windigo (Wiitigo as he refers to it), ideas which were to form the psychiatric idea of Windigo Psychosis, had ever met a victim of the cannibal monster or obtained credible and detailed information about such victims. This was, in Kleinman's terms, a foremost categorical error.

What Parker provides as 'credible' evidence (he also has not met a victim in the flesh) is an elaborate psychoanalytic analysis. For him, when an individual faces a major failure then that person undergoes a sense of worthlessness. He provides the pertinent example of the personal disaster of the hunter not finding food to feed his family as seems to have happened with Swift Runner. When this occurs then:

> [T]he dam (constituted by ego defences) is shattered and the repressed cravings for the expression of dependency and aggressive needs burst forth … [T]he psychotic symptoms serve … to allay dependency cravings (by becoming one with the object of dependency) and to aggress against this frustrating object (by killing and eating it).
>
> *Parker, 1960, p.620*

Parker, however, reinforces the psychiatric explanation that he is criticising for being ill-informed by declaring that in all probability when the 'dam bursts' what transpires is a cultural variation of schizophrenia.

Just a story

Psychologist and anthropologist James Waldram is damning of the disciplines of anthropology and psychiatry as well as psychology for, in his view, producing a distorted portrait of aboriginal peoples. He suggests that members of these assumed intelligent tribes of anthropology, psychiatry and psychology have over decades if not centuries made comparisons and come to conclusions about First Nation tribes, including those in Canada, based on shaky conceptual assumptions, deficient data and stereotyping if not racism. Most, he points out as does Parker, have not met or if they have they have not comprehended the people they are studying. Waldram has spent considerable time with Cree and Ojibwa peoples and portends that this means he understands them better than his intellectual colleagues. What those amongst the Algonquians he met told him was that the Windigo was indeed 'just a story'. Moreover, Waldram mentions another enlightened anthropologist, Lou Marano who had examined the research and theories on Windigo Psychosis, and had already 'dissected' the notion. Marano's dissection had laid bare the erroneousness of the Windigo as a real entity and shown that it only existed as such in the minds of 'gullible' anthropologists:

> Windigo psychosis may well be the most perfect example of the construction of an Aboriginal mental disorder by the scholarly professions, and its persistence dramatically underscores how constructions of the aboriginal by these professions have, like Frankenstein's monster, taken on a life of their own.
>
> *Waldram, 2004, p.18*

What Waldram, again agreeing with Marano, argues is that the story of the Windigo Monster built-up into what began to appear to be a real phenomenon only after the Algonquians had hundreds years of contact with Europeans. It was this contact, argues Waldram, which traumatised the Cree and Ojibwa, and one consequence of this socially produced trauma was what became construed as Windigo Psychosis. Accusations of Windigo were made amongst the Algonquians in order to stigmatise and ostracise individuals who were perceived to be socially deviant. The technique of scapegoating assists groups to restore their security and affirm their identity especially when external forces are a threat to their way of life and possibly their existence. What the naïve anthropologists and psychiatrists mistook for a display of mental disorder, therefore, was the outcome of functional victimisation caused not by individual pathology but collective fear.

Although reassured that the conundrum of the Windigo had been clarified, Waldrum was left with a concern not only about the standing of knowledge in the study of cross-cultural mental disorder. He asks might not the whole of psychiatry's monolithic manual of mental disorders contain many faux-monsters?

> If scholars of both anthropology and psychiatry had been mistaken for so long, what other errors might we have made? Were there more faux-cannibal-psychotic-monsters out there?
>
> *Waldram, 2004, p.5*

Communal drama

Although he may not have met an Algonquian from James Bay, one member of the scholarly professions, Roland Littlewood (2002), Professor of Anthropology and Psychiatry at University College London (Helman's academic home), does appear to have Waldram's wisdom. Littlewood (2002) like Waldram gazes beyond prior assumptions concerning aboriginal people. Littlewood asks if there may be a connection between an individual's susceptibility to mental disorder and wider social adjustments and impositions.

Referring to spirit possession generally and Windigo Psychosis specifically, Littlewood suggests that the possessed individual may not have a 'personal' disorder as such but is (unconsciously) acting out a drama on behalf of his/her community. What Littlewood argues is that in situations of exploitation and subordination outside of Western society madness can emerge in forms relevant to those who are being exploited and subordinated and to the outside imposition on that culture. This for him helps to explain the cannibalistic Windigo becoming more than a folk-tale amongst the Algonquian. It is the communal stress on the Algonquians caused by colonisation that becomes expressed through the exaggeration of an available narrative with violent and vengeful overtones.

The problem with Waldram's and Littlewood's assumptions about social causation is that if Windigo was 'just a story', an accusation, or 'only in the minds' of the gullible, then there could be no social causation because there was no credence given by the Cree to the Windigo either as a reality or metaphor. Moreover, no definitive case of Windigo Psychosis let alone a Windigo psychotic case of cannibalism ever came to light and if exploitation and subordination were such significant catalysts then presumably more Cree would have yielded to this madness or similar exotic ethnic curiosities.

The problem with Helman's and Kleinman's 'biology-plus-society' approach is that the medical understanding of madness can be credible (or regain credibility) if inculcated with a compassion for cultural contexts rather than an acceptance of the possibility that the medicalisation of madness could be displaced by a different perspective, or different society insane or not.

Summary

Utilising the sociological and anthropological ideas of Fromm, Helman, and Kleinman, and a variety of other societally/culturally-minded thinkers I have suggested that Fry's performance as a manic-depressive, celebrity, and alleged (by himself and others) narcissist, and Swift Runner's as a cannibalistic mass murderer, cannot be viewed in isolation from the relevant social context – mature/postmodern capitalism for Fry and colonial Canada for Swift Runner. Manic-depression, celebrity-seeking, normal-narcissism and Windigo Psychosis, therefore become expressions of their respective cultures. Colonisation and environmental hardship in the Cree community fomented the repertoire of a cannibalistic monster but which was serviced by the availability of a draft script from that community's folk-law. Celebrity, narcissism, consumerism, commodification, mass media and biological reductionism, in Westernised communities provide the antecedent script for the repertoire for such mental disorders as manic-depression. Fry and Swift Runner are both perhaps possessed, one by the spirit of capitalism the other by that of a monster.

The logic of Fromm's argument and that emanating from medical anthropology is that if the colonisation of North America had never happened, or if it had not been so culturally overbearing, then there would be no or few instances of mad murderous cannibalism, and if today's (Westernised) society were to change to become sane, the same may come to be said of narcissism and manic-depression.

However, to consider Fry or Swift Runner (or anyone) as sheer casualties of their culture, thereby irreproachable victims, is not sustainable logically. Why is it that these individuals in particular become famous or infamous, and sad, mad or bad? What else is involved which pushes an individual to the forefront of egotism or iniquity? To contrive a phrase and one which I accept seems oxymoronic, are they 'duplicitous-dupes'? As with most humans, Fry and Swift Runner's freedom to think, feel and act is in a reflexive relationship with their societal situation.

Individuals are to some degree masters/mistresses of their own fate but a fate which is conditional on how their society operates. How society operates is conditional on what individuals, either separately or grouped, decide to think, feel and act. Individual volition and societal pressure are in a push-and-pull myriad of complex arrangements which it is problematic to untangle. When the structure of that society is massively and manifestly unjust then the pulls and pushes will be preferential for some and disadvantaging for many. When the ideology of society recommends materialism, celebrity and narcissism, and makes a mental disorder fashionable, then insanity sits outside the individual.

Moreover, individuals are also involved in a similarly multifaceted interplay with the various constituents of their biology and psychology. Some people do manage to escape from the chains of their social system and act, feel, and think differently from the 'insane' inculcations of society. Some people will, become mad no matter what the structure and ideology of society. That is, a sane society is not a cure-all for all insanity.

Notes

1 Unless otherwise referenced details relating to Swift Runner's life and performance have been extracted from Thomson (1984) and in particular the Library and Archives Canada (1994); media sources have also been used to triangulate 'facts', many of which are listed in Thomson.

Further reading

Fromm, F. (1955) *The Sane Society*. New York: Rinehart.

Helman, C. (2007) (fifth edition) *Culture, Health and Illness*. London: Hodder Arnold.

Liddle, R. (2014) *Selfish Whining Monkeys: How We Ended Up Greedy, Narcissistic and Unhappy*. London: Fourth Estate.

Waldram, J. (2004) *Revenge of the Windigo: The Construction of the Mind and Mental Health of North American Aboriginal Peoples*. Toronto: University of Toronto Press.

5

SCIENCE AND PSYCHIATRY

Susannah Cahalan

Susannah Cahalan (*circa* 1985–) thought she had bed bugs. She had not, but she was heading towards probable coma and possible death passing first through a wide range of serious psychological and physiological symptoms, a million dollars' worth of medical tests, disengaged identity and ultimately a self-declared change in personhood.

Cahalan (2012a) has written a best-selling autobiographical book about how during 2009 at the age of 24 years she experienced what she describes as her 'month of madness'. Amongst the multitude of medical diagnoses made about this mad month were the psychotic conditions of manic-depression, schizophrenia and schizoaffective disorder, which is schizophrenia and manic-depression combined. However, the numbness, fluctuating heart rate, and in particular the seizures she suffered stood out as symptoms not usually associated with such psychiatric diagnoses. Nor did the result of a simple and cost-free 'clock test' which was to indicate that she was not at root experiencing madness.

An award-winning journalist who works for the *New York Post*, Cahalan used her memory and journalistic skills to research the events leading-up to, within, and following her 'month of madness'. She appreciated, however, that her autobiographical narrative would inevitably be contaminated by subjectivity (as are all autobiographies and much of journalism), and by what she admits were her severe mental impediments at the time of her supposed madness (2012a). To reduce partiality and muddling, she conducted hundreds of interviews with the doctors and nurses with whom she had contact and examined thousands of pages of documents associated with her case as well as the videos of her taken whilst she was hospitalised. Moreover, to be better informed, she studied the various conditions voiced as her presumed or suspected diagnosis. Furthermore, her own contemporaneous notes, along with those made by her divorced parents whilst she was being handled – or rather mishandled – by those employed in the psychiatric system and other health arenas, were scrutinised (Cahalan, 2012b; 2013).

Historical resonances

Cahalan's contact with the medical profession in the twenty-first century has particular parallels with that undergone by the John Perceval in the nineteenth century (see Chapter 2) and Mary Barnes in the twentieth century (see Chapter 2). Over 170 years after Perceval's encounter with doctors and attendants and their manacles, and over 70 years since Barnes was put in a padded-cell, Cahalan was similarly restrained. This time, however, it is the medical and nursing staff within a general hospital setting where Cahalan has been admitted after becoming confused and unconscious that utilises physical control. She awakes to find that she is restrained:

> My fingers find a thick mesh vest at my waist holding me to the bed like a … straightjacket. The vest connects to two cold metal rails. I wrap my hands around the rails and pull up, but again the straps dig into my chest, yielding only a few inches.
>
> *Cahalan, 2012a, p.xi*

The fettering of Cahalan was employed by hospital staff to prevent her hurting herself from, for example, falling out of bed. The threat of self-injury and causing injury to others, accepted as factual by Cahalan (2012b; 2013), resulted in the administering of sedative medication. Justifying the necessity does not detract, however, from the controlling nature of these interventions. In essence, what happened to Cahalan does not differ either in intent or content from what Perceval underwent in a nineteenth century asylum or Barnes in a twentieth century mental hospital. In all three cases, medical authority superseded personal autonomy.

Furthermore, the disagreements between medical professionals over Cahalan's diagnosis echo those disputing the precise cause of Pierre Rivière's homicidal performance two centuries later (see Chapter 1). Whilst Cahalan did not kill anyone her psycho-somatic symptomatology exposes the medical profession's continued querulousness over correct categorisation even when the patient is demonstrating raw and arrant indications of malady.

Over 170 years after debates amongst the medical profession about the psychological condition of Rivière, Cahalan experiences similar medical diagnostic turpitude but covering a much wider list of possible complaints from a far larger group of medical practitioners. Apart from manic-depression, schizophrenia and schizoaffective disorder, she was suspected to be suffering from alcoholism; anxiety; attention-seeking; mononucleosis; a form of compulsive-obsessive disorder (parasitosis or Ekhom syndrome where fear of obsession of infestation leads to a preoccupation with cleaning); epilepsy; teratoma; Capgras syndrome (hallucinations and delusions directed towards family members); postictal psychosis (seizures and later delusions, hallucinations, mood changes including aggressiveness); multiple/dissociative personality disorder; and depression.

All of these suspected disorders turned out to be wrong or symptomatic of another primary diagnosis. Those who provide an opinion included: Cahalan's gynaecologist who was also her friend; two eminent neurologists, accident-emergency department junior doctors; two psychiatrists; approximately nine non-eminent neurologists; a psycho-pharmacologist; a neurosurgeon; a neurologist who eventually became esteemed in the fields of neuropathology and epileptology.

As demonstrated markedly in Rosenhan's (1973) studies, discussed in Chapter 3, diagnostic uncertainty has haunted psychiatry throughout its history. However, unlike the one-off voices of Rosenhan's participants, Cahalan presented with many disparate symptoms: fearfulness; free-floating anxiety; irrational jealousy; weeping; insomnia; despair; grunting; nightmares; impulsiveness; agoraphobia; feelings of persecution; belief that her father was an imposter; confusion; nausea and vomiting; headache; loss of appetite; pins and needles and numbness; thrusting her arm forward involuntarily; tongue lolling; grimacing; urinary incontinence; and seizures. Hence, diagnostic certainty would have been miraculous certainly if attained at an early stage. Many basic and sophisticated tests to find the probable diagnosis and differential diagnoses were carried out. These included blood analyses, computerised tomography (CT), magnetic resonance imaging (MRI), positron emission tomography (PET), electro-encephalogram and a brain biopsy. Rosenhan's participants were largely assessed through sketchy surveillance and infrequent consultation. Also, to be fair to those of her doctors who considered Cahalan mad, the list of symptoms, most of which were mental in presentation or could reasonably be suspected of being mental in origin, would understandably lead them at least initially to that conclusion. Those which were not might excusably be judged as psycho-somatic, that is the physical presentation of a mental disorder.

Dalmau's disease

Cahalan was eventually diagnosed after moving from medical practitioner to medical practitioner, and medical facility to medical facility, by the above mentioned neurologist who was to become a venerated neuropathologist and epileptologist. That neurologist, Souhel Najjir, judged that Cahalan had an exceptional and potentially fatal autoimmune disorder affecting proteins in the nerve cell receptors on the surface of the brain. The indication that this might be the cause of Cahalan's 'month of madness' arose from Najjir asking her to take the 'Clock Drawing Test', which has gained the reputation as an ideal preliminary check on cognitive ability. As a screening instrument, it could not be simpler. The patient is merely asked to draw a clock with the numbers placed correctly. If there is cognitive impairment then it is likely to be drawn incorrectly (Shulman, 2000). Cahalan placed the numbers only on one side of the clock and was unaware that she had done so.

Moreover, the results of the subsequent brain biopsy ordered by Najjir revealed inflammation and encephalitis. Najjar reasoned that the probable cause of her psychological and physical symptoms is a type of encephalitis which has the technical name of 'anti-N-methyl-D-aspartic acid receptor encephalitis' (Dalmau's Disease). Najjar explained less technically to Cahalan and her parents:

> Her [Cahalan] brain is on fire … Her brain is under attack from her own body.
>
> *Najjar in Cahalan, 2012, p. 134*

The implications of this diagnosis for Najjar are immense. Najjar is reported by Cahalan in her book (2012a) to believe that inflammation of the brain is the cause of manic-depression, obsessive-compulsive disorder, depression and schizophrenia. In a later publication Najjar focuses on the latter and states his belief in the possibilities that neurology[1] can offer to understanding this disorder:

> If an autoimmune disease can create symptoms that look exactly like schizophrenia, that raises the question, what is schizophrenia? And are there forms of schizophrenia that are caused by other types of autoimmune disease? Or other [physical] diseases that we haven't discovered yet? **It's all neurological**. [emphases added]
>
> *Najjar quoted in Cadwalladr, 2013*

Increasingly, immunological disturbances, many of which induce inflammation in the central nervous system, are linked to a wide range of mental disorders. Examples of such disorders include schizophrenia, depression, obsessive-compulsive disorder, Alzheimer's disease, and *Gilles de la Tourette's* syndrome (World Psychiatric Association, 2015b). Immuno-psychiatry,[2] a subdivision of molecular psychiatry, is proposed by some psychiatrists orientated to neuroscience to be nothing less than a radically new science of the mind (Schwartz, 2010; Bullmore quoted in Gallagher *et al.*, 2016).

Once Cahalan was diagnosed with Dalmau's Disease her treatment regime shifted from being anti-insanity to anti-inflammatory: intravenous and then oral steroids. Any permanent damage to the brain caused by such pathology as encephalitis may be over-ridden by encouraging 'neurogenesis'. That is, it is possible that brain function could be regained and madness founded in neuropathology resolved through the growth of new brain tissue, undamaged neurons forming new pathways, or neurological activity 'assembling' differently (Inta *et al.*, 2016; Greenfield, 2016). Neuroplasticity with respect to cognitive ability can be encouraged, as it was to aid Cahalan's memory and ability to think rationally, through psychological interventions (Cahalan, 2012a).

The proposition that many mental disorders are caused by neurological disturbances, immunologically inflammatory or not, seems to underscore Szasz's idea (see Chapter 3) that if there is no neurological pathology present then mental disorder is a myth. If there is a neurological pathology then it is not a mental disorder but neurological disorder, and to be dealt with by neurologists not psychiatrists of any hue. However, psychiatry in the main appears to be striving to embrace neuroscience, not to dissolve into a neuroscientific sub-branch (White *et al.*, 2012).

Tenacity and resources

Cahalan points out that had not it been for her tenacity and social skills and the unremitting support of her family and boyfriend, along with the financial funding received from her medical insurance company to pay for her prolonged and disabling afflictions and associated medical escapades, she may have spent years in an institution if not the rest of her life:

> I think about, I can't help but think about all those people out there throughout history who went undiagnosed, misdiagnosed, overlooked, I think about people who were put in psychiatric hospitals, I think about people who were given exorcisms, I can't help but think about all those people, and I think about how lucky I was, how extremely lucky I was to meet a man [Najjar] who thought outside the box.
>
> *Cahalan, 2013*

Cahalan continues with her journalistic career and family life. She uses the success of her book to raise awareness about her condition and to expose her medical misadventures through misdiagnosis. Her story has been repeated in various news-media articles and in the professional press (Cadwalladr, 2013; Costello, 2014). There are also video recordings in which she tells of her story and these can be accessed by the public via the Internet. One of the recordings is of her lecture for the organisation set up to disseminate ideas, 'TED' (Cahalan, 2013). Moreover, there is a film in preparation telling her story (Broadgreen Pictures, 2016).

Cahalan is *de facto* a 'psychiatric survivor' in the sense of having been rescued from psychiatry by neurology. But, neurology may be crucial to the rescuing of psychiatry.

Peter McGuffin and Stephen Rose

Can a 'revitalised' and more scientific psychiatry infused with and enthused by the empirical outpourings of neuroscience and those of genetic research, together with the associated diagnostic technologies and physical methods of treatment (drugs, brain surgery, and molecular manipulation, and a few 'evidence-based' psychotherapies) secure the future of psychiatry? This proposition formed a debate involving psychiatrist and geneticist Peter McGuffin, at that time director of the social, genetic and development psychiatry centre at King's College London, and neurobiologist Steven Rose,[3] then director of the brain and behaviour research group at the Open University (Rose and McGuffin, 2005). The article logging their debate is titled 'Will Science Explain Mental Illness?'

McGuffin's stance is that brain imaging and molecular genetics offer much scientific promise for psychiatry. He points out that specific areas of the human brain can be observed to 'light up' using MRI when intellectual and emotional tasks are performed. This type of in-depth imaging can show neurological 'functional' changes rather than just lesions when the subject is experiencing hallucinations or delusions, and drugs can reverse some these brain aberrations. Studies of twins and people adopted indicate that inheritance is significant in the cause of serious mental disorder. Sets of genes implicated in the cause of schizophrenia and manic-depression have been identified, and the responsible mix of faulty genes for many other disorders will eventually be found and fixed.

Rose responds by accepting that neurology and genetics have to be considered with regard to 'psychic distress'. However, it is, he explains, axiomatic that psychological states have corresponding brain states. That is a person who is, for example, psychotic will have different brain processes and therefore dissimilar brain images to those of someone who is not experiencing delusions or hallucinations. Furthermore, giving drugs which alter the patient's neuro-chemistry will, of course, alter his/her performance. But, argues Rose, imaging only provides evidence of association not proof of origin. Moreover, he repeats what has been claimed by, for example Richard Bentall (see Chapter 3), that it is only the surface presentation of a supposed disorder which is affected by drugs, not the would- be source, and even when medication is 'effective' this does not confirm that the root of mental disorder is biological. He offers the following comparator to illustrate his reasoning:

> [A]spirin alleviates the pain of toothache, but we don't conclude that the cause of toothache is too little aspirin in the brain.
>
> *Rose in Rose and McGuffin, 2005, p.30*

Rose is another advocate of listening to patients rather than allowing technology and physical methods to resolve the patient's psychological predicaments. The psychiatrist, and by implication any other clinician with a professional leaning towards neuroscience and genetics and their concomitant ingesting, implanting and editing therapies, should be open to 'hear' the patient's story and allow that story to dictate the terms of assessment and remedy (Rose in Rose and McGuffin, 2005).

Continuing his attack not just on McGuffin's position but that of all psychiatrists who are orientated to biology, Rose argues that a fundamental flaw in their reasoning is that they attempt to measure scientifically what is not defined adequately by them or indeed what is not definable at all. What, he asks, is the borderline between anxiety and depression, or schizophrenia and manic-depression? He notes the cases of patients who regularly have their diagnosis transmuted between these categories and consequently their treatments vary. The highly precise instruments of neuroscience and genetics are being applied to highly imprecise psychiatric labels. McGuffin's response is that rather than abandoning these technologies and diagnoses, the science behind them and their connectedness needs to be advanced.

Biology acknowledges Rose, is certainly involved in some conditions such as Alzheimer's Disorder. But, Rose suggests that there is abundant evidence of psycho-social development tribulations and unfortunate social factors such as poverty, poor housing and familial discord, having as much if not more impact on mental disorder overall than neurological and genetic mishap. This leads Rose to the conclusion that the answer to mental disorder may not lie with science.

This debate between McGuffin and Rose opens-up three core questions concerning science and psychiatry. These are: what are the properties of scientific knowledge? How robust and relevant is psychiatric science based on neuroscience and genetics? Might a synthesis of different forms of knowledge be more appropriate for understanding and managing madness?

Scientific fundamentals

In Westernised and Westernising countries, scientific knowledge and its concomitant technologies are promulgated as the pinnacle epistemology. The stance of science is that only it can furnish verifiable facts and dissemble falsehoods. For science historian Michael Shermer (2015) scientific scepticism about what can be claimed as authentic knowledge, which for him can only be that which relies on rationalism and empiricism, is the driving force behind making humans much more moral than religion or other systems of thought such as those arising from religion and political ideology.

However, competing ways of comprehending the natural and social world as well the conceiving of transcendental existences abound. Despite thousands of years of scientific epistemological insurgency, religion, superstition, folklore, new-ageism, experientialism, intuition, inanity and insanity co-exist with the laws of physics, chemistry, biology, mathematics, cosmology and their equivalents within social science. Moreover, some varieties of sociological thinking have challenged the authenticity and authority of any epistemology to claim access to truth and reality.

Notable advocates of science are Lewis Wolpert (2000), Emeritus Professor of Developmental Biology, University College, London; Richard Dawkins (2006), Professor of the Public Understanding of Science at Oxford University; Steven Pinker (2013), Professor of Psychology at Harvard University and Ben Goldacre (2009), British-trained medical practitioner. Dawkins, Wolpert, Pinker and Goldacre, regard science as the only way to understand natural and social phenomena. Moreover, they are science evangelists. They advocate the vigorous dissemination of scientific rules and results throughout society. Scientifically-verified rational thinking, politics and social policies for them are crucial for the generation of a civilised society. Rational thought founded on science should also underpin human morality.

These evangelising scientists assail what in their view are the abuses of science and the threats to rational thinking and rational morality. These include: the use of scientific discoveries for warfare; the post-modern position that everything and nothing is believable; supposed-scientific data presented in the popular media to give credence to a range of advice about lifestyle and health, and to back political campaigns and policies; the manipulation of scientific data to sell medical products, especially pharmaceuticals; religion of all hues but especially those espousing fundamentalist beliefs. They fear the swamping of society with asinine, and unconstructive if not destructive thinking and customs. What for them is needed for society to progress is more critical analyses and constructive answers from science about such social problems as poverty, global warming and disease.

Wolpert, Dawkins, Pinker and Goldacre's version of science is attuned to the notion of intellectual and innovative progression from the Ancient Greco-Roman Empires onwards. The ancient Greeks, who themselves received ideas from previous civilisations such as those of the Babylonians and Egyptians, had methodically studied medicine, astronomy, cosmology, geometry, mathematics, electricity, magnetism, human biology, zoology and geography. The Romans added engineering and technology to the knowledge of the Greeks and extended medical knowledge. Myth, however, overshadowed the embryonic scientific thinking of the Greeks and the Romans (Lindberg, 1992).

Belief in superstition and the celestial ascended during the European Dark-Ages and Middle-Ages. The hegemony of the Roman Catholic Church meant that having non-religious (that is non-Christian) thoughts about how the world and universe worked could bring about accusations of heresy which might then lead to torture and execution (Lambert, 2002). The danger of death for improper thinking did not fully displace Greek and Roman science in Europe. However, the humanism of the Renaissance (fourteenth to the seventeenth century) began to undermine religion and a torrent of new ways of thinking emerged which focused on questioning assumptions about nature and society including those held by the Ancients.

In the seventeenth century rationalism, along with human liberty, was a key element of the European Enlightenment (Burnett, 2015). The mantles of 'The Scientific Revolution' given to that period and then the 'The Age-of-Reason' in the eighteenth century indicate a major shift away from the ideological control of the Church and the naïveté of Greco-Roman science. Voltaire (1694–1778) campaigned against injustice, intolerance and bigotry, and René Descartes (1596–1650) generated ideas that led to the foundation of modern philosophy and mathematics. Francis Bacon's (1561–1626) favouring of empirical observation as the *sin qua non* of scientific method continues to be influential today. Nicolaus Copernicus (1473–1543) calculation of positions of the planets and his pronouncement that the earth revolved around the sun: Galilei Galileo (1564–1642) gauging that objects with unlike mass will fall at the same rate, and his designing of an effective telescope. Sir Isaac Newton (1642–1727) formulated laws of gravitational force, calculus, optics and motion, and along with the sociologist Auguste Comte (1798–1857) – a version of science known as 'positivism'.

Sociologist Gerard Delanty (1997) lists the core tenets of positivistic science:

a   empiricism – we only know what can be observed;
b   experiment is the basis of scientific observation as it can reveal cause-and-effect relationships;
c   all knowledge is susceptible to the techniques of natural science;
d   there is a reality which can be studied, and science stands;
    objectively and value-free outside this reality;
e   internally coherent and universal laws exist and cross-over bodies of knowledge.

Positivism was to provide the intellectual nutrients for the gestation and sustaining of myriad technical innovations which were to fuel the industrial revolution of the eighteenth and nineteenth centuries. Moreover, science and technology were inexorably connected with capitalist expansion globally, and which by the middle of the twentieth century was to encompass both manufacturing and service industries.

What positivism also posits is that any ideas outside that realm of science would be pure fantasy or fallacy. That is, only knowledge produced and tested by science can claim to be truthful and real (Burnett, 2015).

However, positivism was to undergo modification in the twentieth century. What led to this modification and its consequences can be observed by examining what became known as the 'Popper-Kuhn Debate'. This debate centred on the question of what can be counted as real and truthful in science.

Popper and Kuhn

On one side of the debate was Sir Karl Popper, a philosopher of science who argued for a particular version of scientific purism which narrowed considerably the scope of science to claim to be seeking or to have found proven facts. On the other side was science historian Thomas Kuhn who, whilst not antagonistic to science, reasoned that it could never be 'pure' because its organisation and principles were influenced inevitably and extensively by the epoch and culture in which it occurred as well as by the psychology of scientists.

For Popper (1959), science should not be set-up to establish definite and consistent truths. In his view, such a goal was impossible to achieve except in rare circumstances. Scientific endeavour was doomed to failure and derision if it continued to maintain, in the positivistic sense, that provable facts had been or would be found to explain reality and truth. Popper argued that science instead should be founded on falsification. That is, scientific research should only attempt to find 'false' correlations between events or phenomena. To conjecture that 'all swans are white' because all of the swans observed so far (that is, through the collection of empirical data) have been white is vulnerable to failure as a fact because it doesn't allow for the possibility of discovering one black swan.

The contention that particular mental disorders are caused by synaptic misconfigurations, malformed genes, bio-chemical imbalance or brain anatomical anomalies cannot be sustained as a Popperian scientific proposition. Apart from a known number of issues concerning sample sizes and circular reasoning which indicate the tenuousness of these biological causative connections, the existence of one person (let alone most people) with any of these disorders having a 'normal' biology causes the fact to fail. Equally, the occurrence of one person with one of these biological deviations who does not have a mental disorder.

What Popper wanted was the formulation of scientific questions which from the outset were trying to disprove relationships between variables (for example, apples and acceleration, mental disorder and faulty biology, whiteness and swans). Questions which could not be framed for falsification lay, he argued, outside the remit of science. If a proposition cannot be proven wrong, then this is not science he argued. 'Does God exist'? is not a scientific question for Popper as the existence of God depends on belief and in any case cannot be tested by any methodical means within science to-date. Establishing a hard-and-fast fusion between the Freudian notions of structures of the mind (the id, ego and superego) and an individual's behaviour is inherently problematic for Popper's idea of science. Freud's id, ego and superego are abstracts and thereby cannot be proven to not exist (or exist). Behaviour is concrete and can be measured and tested for falsification. Moreover, testing a relationship between the abstract and the concrete is futile. The 'null hypothesis' based on testing a non-connection becomes one way of enacting the principle of falsification. For example, it is logically feasible to come to the conclusion that there is no association between smoking and cancer – although of course there is a mass of evidence to support the hypothesis that smoking does cause cancer.

However, the positivist view of scientific advancement as a relentless journey towards finding truth and reality and the logical positivist interjection that the route of science should be one which steers away from falsehoods was challenged by Kuhn (1962). Kuhn's position is that during long periods of what he termed 'normal science' scientists merely accepted or possibly modified mildly the presumptions of their predecessors. Scientists in these periods operate within an overarching paradigm of thought handed down by those in the scientific field who had become established as experts, that is those whose work had attracted substantial funding and had been published in high-reputation journals. These prestigious scientists founded the field of knowledge relevant to their subject, and for the most part, their colleagues merely addressed particular puzzles that were internal to their specialist sub-paradigm or tinkered with its parameters. Only those problems to be funded and then researched, and the only conclusions sanctioned and disseminated, are those that are plausible to the paradigm. Any thinking or evidence that springs up during the 'normal science' period which seems to contradict the precepts of the paradigm are ignored or disposed through ridicule or snubbing. Another protective technique to ensure the continuation of the paradigm's legitimacy is the designing of theories and the finding of associative evidence paradigmatically synchronised. For Kuhn, the scientific community, therefore, was usually self-indoctrinating and self-perpetuating. The normal period of science was indulgent not expectant, raising its own brood of ideas and data not gestating intellectual and evidential cuckoos.

However, Kuhn introduced a radical idea into his thinking about the character of science, and one which has much continued importance. What Kuhn pointed out is that at various times in the history of science there is such a build-up of ideas and evidence contrary to that which fits with what has become the conventional scientific way of viewing the natural and social world, that the legitimacy of the normal paradigm starts to collapse. This for Kuhn heralds an era of 'revolutionary science'. The hegemony of 'normal' scientific disintegrates, and the old truths and realities cannot be sustained. Turmoil within the scientific community ensues until innovative truths and realities can make sense of the new 'facts' as they unfold through further research and theorising. Then the whole circle of normalising scientific discovery followed eventually by the interceding of abnormal scientific findings repeat. The replacement paradigm may or may not be an improvement on previous paradigms. There is no guarantee, suggests Kuhn, of scientific progress as such, only irregular seismic shifts in what is considered progressive.

Kuhn also points out that what counts as scientific data in the positivist tradition is that which can be separated from 'theory'. Empirical evidence should be collected objectively and this should be so whether research is deductive (theory-testing) or inductive (theory-crafting). However, facts cannot actually be collected objectively as any observation is already contaminated, or 'theory-laden', by the views and practices of the scientific paradigm's architects and their disciples. This may seem like a postmodernist deconstructionist approach, which renders science nothing more than one possible system of belief out of limitless contenders. Understanding that science is not value-free is not the same as arguing it has no value or as much value as a belief in an all-powerful creator and creationism. It does, however, challenge the positivists' avowal that good science is insuperably accurate (Burnett, 2015).

Black swans make an appearance again in scholar and statistician Nassim Taleb's (2006) book appropriately titled *Black Swan*. He argues that science privileges its own knowledge to convince itself and try to convince everyone that the universe and everything it is understandable and therefore predictable or has the potential so to be with further research by scientists. The proclaimed robustness of its techniques and laws is founded, however, on the trick of forming the rules and concepts which allow such substantiation. Efficacy professed by science is 'epistemological arrogance' suggests Taleb. The natural and the social world is much more prone to random happenings akin to the appearance of the allegorical 'black swan' in a world in which the illusion has been recorded by science that all swans are white. For Taleb, there is a 'great intellectual fraud' occurring whereby certainty is promulgated rather than uncertainty being admitted to be the driving force of scientific and social change. The Black Swan incidents should be embraced, humans should get far more excited by and reliant upon the unknowable rather than the knowable.

> This implies that we need to use the extreme event as a starting point and not treat it as an exception to be pushed under the rug.
>
> *Taleb, 2006, p.xxviii*

Scientific flakiness

That science is affected by extraneous factors is well known. What is studied, how it is studied and which results are disseminated, depend in the main on finding funds. Finding the funds to carry-out research depends on the interests of the funding provider (Goldacre, 2012). Moreover, political interference may arise especially when governmental departments are supplying the funds. For example, British senior scientists who receive government grants reported that they feared that results from their research which may not favour policies advocated by the politically powerful would not be allowed to be published (Wilsdon and Main, 2016). This fear is associated with the trend by British governments to insist that any research it funds has practical and immediate utility thereby reducing the potential for 'blue skies' ideas to emerge which may be of academic interest but may in the future have practical use.

A key factor in the claim of scientific robustness is the implementation of 'peer review'. Sense about Science (2016), the pro-science lobby group, hallows peer review as the most objective way of assessing the value of research and thereby allowing publication of the findings in what are known in academic jargon as 'high-impact' journals. Virtually all such journals are committed to the peer review process to legitimate their publications. But, the selection of reviewers is a prejudiced process – made by editors or recommended by other reviewers. Moreover, the selected and the selectors are already part of normal science. Far from being objective, peer review can be viewed as a pooling of subjectivity (Morrall, 2009).

John Ioannidis (2005; 2014) Professor of Medicine and Professor of Statistics at Stanford University records that approximately 5 million scientific papers are published annually by about 3 million authors in academic and professional journals. However, Ioannidis claims the vast majority of the findings from the studies on which the material for these papers is drawn are exaggerated or false. This includes research appertaining to the biological basis of madness, notably neurological findings. The exaggeration and falseness occurs because of fundamental faults in the design of the studies, especially a narrowness in sample selection, definitional and methodological 'flexibility', and a lack of statistical power for the analysis. There is also, argues Ioannidis, considerable as well as inherent bias due to the personal prejudices and financial interests of the researchers and other stakeholders. Ioannidis suggests that biomedical research is replete with these conflicts of interest and this is in part because this type of research is highly popular. Few indisputable and applicable advances are made from this mass of scientific endeavour.

For unorthodox scientist Rupert Sheldrake (2012), the 'delusion' of science is the narrowness of its gaze. Science, argues Sheldrake, has focused on human inquisitiveness far too much for far too long on material questions and answers. Alternative, metaphysical, transcendental, telepathic and 'psychic' conundrums and resolutions should be considered equally valid as perspectives to understand people and the physical and social environment.

Furthermore, science cannot avoid contamination by political and public opinion which may also concern questions of morality. Whether it is global warming, atom bombs, conventional weaponry, abortion, hybrid human-animal embryos, pan-industrialisation or migration, science is caught in a maze of ethical dilemmas. Any refusal by scientists and scientific organisations to opine on morality does not negate or delegate the moral/immoral consequence of scientific research.

For biologist Brian Goodwin (2007) scientific knowledge can only ever be an interpretation of reality. He accepts that subjective views and social processes interfere with the search for facts. Goodwin's solution is the formation of a new culturally-sensitive and holistic science, which understands these interferences. Attempting to unite all of the scientific disciplines and sensitise their endeavours with the vast array of understandings gleaned from the copious numbers of cultures across the world (accepting that many have become consumed by the values and practices of capitalism) seems somewhat idealistic. Philosopher Simon Blackburn (2006) argues that the search by scientists for truth and reality is a laudable and valuable pursuit, but that scepticism should be adopted not only by scientists but also about science ever attaining this goal.

The history of science is not one of simple progression or recognisable revolutionary transformation. Science stutters, backtracks, jumps forward haphazardly, plausibly, serendipitously, as well as in great-leaps, and at times surpasses, overtakes, accompanies, complements or contends with other epistemologies (Gribbin, 2003).

> In the sphere of thought, sober civilisation is roughly synonymous with science. But science unadulterated, is not satisfying; men [and women] need also passion and art and religion. Science may set limits to knowledge, but should not set limits to imagination.
>
> *Russell, 1961, p.36*

Ironically, the temporal standing of science as the foremost epistemology is implied in a newspaper article written by Venki Ramakrishnan, current president of the Royal Society. The Royal Society is a prestigious scientific academy founded in the seventeenth century with a mandate to deliver the message that science is both effective and beneficial for society. Ramakrishnan asks the readership to imagine travelling back 200 years to explain to the intellectual elite of that time that in future centuries humans would be able to decode the locus of heredity, to know how humanity had evolved, to have obtained details about how the universe began, to have found out that physical properties at the sub-molecular level act counter to the laws of physics at other levels, to be able to communicate instantaneously across continents, and to cure chronic disease with drugs called antibiotics. The reaction of these ancestors, Ramakrishnan exclaims, would be incredulity:

> They would be in awe of us and think we were magicians.
>
> *Ramakrishnan, 2016*

However, what is also incredible is that Ramakrishnan does not recognise that these ancestors would have been viewed as magicians by their ancestors and that such incredulity could be attributed to future 'magicians' by today's intelligentsia about the way in which physical and social minutiae and totalities have become comprehended.

Scientism and magic

The projection of science as the arbiter of truth and the only repository of what is real is the 'magic' that is conjured particularly by positivists. This discriminatory position regarding what can be counted as genuine knowledge is described as 'scientism'. Scientism is an accusatory attribution which goes beyond the recognition that science is tainted by social processes and the unpredicted arrival of black swans. What the concept of scientism infers is that there an unjustified and exaggerated confidence that science is capable of solving all intellectual questions and all human problems (Robinson and Williams, 2015).

Science is a human practice and a cultural phenomenon which as with all other human practices and cultural phenomena is moulded by subjectivity and contexts. It does not stand outside humanity or society. Scientism infers that the locating of science as the supreme stance on knowing everything and anything is fallacious (Robinson and Williams, 2015). An analogy illustrating this fallacy is offered by science writer Thomas Burnett:

> [T]o claim there is nothing knowable outside the scope of science would be similar to a successful fisherman saying that whatever he can't catch in his nets does not exist Once you accept that science is the only source of human knowledge, you have adopted a philosophical position

(scientism) that cannot be verified, or falsified, by science itself. It is, in a word, unscientific.

Burnett, 2015

However, the idea of scientism is also based on fallacious logic – that of the straw-man.

Straw-man

The 'straw-man' (illogical and self-serving) argument is the erection of a stance which no one actually holds but which then allows the 'challenger' of that stance to assert a particular viewpoint and one which is more than likely already set and possibly fixed to a pre-held ideology.

The actuality of normal science, I suggest, does not fit the model presented by either the purists or their detractors. Science is not a homogenous discipline with a rampant hegemonic praxis, nor has it united through one methodology (falsification or otherwise). If science is a community, then it is a very fractious one with vicious internal feuds, subdivisions, and continuing procedural and epistemological disagreements (Fuller, 2014). Given the complexity of the organic and inorganic spheres, it would be magical if knowledge could be so cultivatable let alone complete. To collect and contain real and truthful understandings of the grand-scale of the universe and the infinitesimal movements of molecules, the orderly laws of gravity and the unruly conduct of the quantum, the habits of the millions of different animal and plant species on earth alone, the structures and processes of globalising society and those appertaining to impersonal communication, would not only be magical but illusory. But that does not mean that science (and technology), including that of medical science, has not made enormous and tangible strides in the direction of the civilised society.

Psychiatric science

The protagonists of science in psychiatry seem undaunted by or unaware of these internal and external criticisms of science in general. For example, Henry Nasralla, Editor in Chief of the journal *Current Psychiatry* in an article in which he professes support for anti-psychiatry because it performs the service to orthodox psychiatry of testing its honesty and rigour, announces the scientific prestige of his profession:

[P]sychiatry has evolved into a major scientific and medical discipline.

Nasralla, 2011

Thomas Insel is director of the US National Institute of Mental Health and a member of the US National Academy of Medicine. He argues that advances in biological research have allowed psychiatry to be reinvented. Psychiatry for

Insel is in a pre-revolutionary state. He claims that the ideological and practical armaments for the impending transformation of psychiatry are the diagnostic and curative bullets being generated by genomics and neuroscience to combat, he cites depression and schizophrenia. Insel is in no doubt that mental disorder is a disorder of the brain and in particular a consequence of 'connectopathies', that is problems in neurological circuits.

Dawkins (2015), the evolutionary biologist, ardent rationalist and atheist, dedicated seller of science, is keen to push the message that mental disorder begins in biology. His excitement is palpable regarding the findings of one genetic study into to what he refers to as 'this devastating psychiatric disease', that is schizophrenia (Richard Dawkins Foundation, 2016). What he is referring to is the genetic analysis of nearly 65,000 people which he hails as a 'landmark' in the search for biological causation. For Dawkins, the study 'changes the game' not only in the search for precise causation but for early detection, effective treatment to deal with the source, not just the symptoms, and possibly prevention. What this study purports to show is that 'synaptic pruning' is key to understanding the risk of contracting schizophrenia. According to the researchers who conducted the study, certain protective connections between neurons are eliminated because of the malfunctioning of a specific gene (Sekar *et al.*, 2016).

Evolutionary psychology

Dawkins owes his intellectual inheritance to Charles Darwin and Alfred Russel Wallace (Darwin and Russel, 1858; Darwin, 1859). Their work kick-started scholarly theorising on the origin of species and natural selection. Evolutionary ideas which focus on how biology influences present human performance owe their origins in large part to the 'sociobiology' of Edward Osborne Wilson (1975). Wilson conceived many of his thoughts about humans from studying ants, an interest he had formed in childhood and one which was to lead to a becoming a celebrated myrmecologist. The contention of the sociobiology thesis is that nature rather than nurture could explain all human traits.

Evolutionary psychology is an offspring of Darwinian evolutionary theory and sociobiology (Buss, 2014). Evolutionary psychologists, and their clinical associate's evolutionary psychiatrists argue that normal and abnormal human performance today stems from the biology of early humans. For the psychological and psychiatric evolutionists of all hues the drive for genetic survival and reproduction is primary to all forms of life, including that of humans:

> Boys are made to squirt and girls are made to lay eggs. And if the truth be known, boys don't very much care what they squirt into. Crude though it may be, Gore Vidal's pithy quote neatly sums up the argument for evolutionary psychology.
>
> *Malik, 1998*

All thoughts, behaviours and emotions are construed by the evolutionary psychologists/psychiatrists as functional or dysfunctional in terms of genetic survival. It may seem that depression, schizophrenia, psychopathy and mania are dysfunctional for the individual and society. Certainly, psychiatry has traditionally taken the professional and state-sponsored approach of attempting to correct or at least contain such apparent dysfunctionality. Counter-intuitively, however, these psychological states may not be maladaptive but adaptive. They may operate at the level of the 'gene' to aid the recovery of the individual from stressful life events and thereby be beneficial to the 'genetic pool' of humanity and potentially society. For example, experiencing miserableness (which might be medicalised as depression) may allow an individual to disengage from the pressures of life and gain an opportunity to recover from disappointment, bereavement or bewilderment. Feelings of unease (potentially attracting a diagnosis of anxiety) about some situations or people afford a psychological signal of possible danger enabling flight or fight preparation. Unusual beliefs and sensations (liable to be medically classifiable as the delusions and hallucinations of schizophrenia) could provide a creative and serviceable perspective to deal with unusual circumstances such as famine, warfare or an apparent anomaly in the laws of normal science. Extravagant egotism and flagrant indifference to the needs of others (psychiatric signs of psychopathy) may be just the type of 'ordered' rather than 'disordered' personality needed to procure mates with whom to propagate or help propagate the profits of global corporations (Stevens and Price, 2000; Brune, 2008; Andrews and Thomson, 2009).

Dawkins (1976) helpfully handed his evolutionary compatriots in psychology and by association that of evolutionary psychiatry the concept of the 'meme' to explain how elements of culture and human performance such as specific rules and ideas about morality might be passed from one generation to another. The meme is meant not to be just a metaphor but have an existence similar to that of a virus (Brodie, 2009). The idea of a biologically-driven conduit for personal and cultural attributes, however, is highly controversial (Rose, 1998). Moreover, there is little hard evidence to back psychology/psychiatry's version of Darwinian biology (Rose and Rose, 2001; Goldacre, 2007; Tallis, 2004, 2014).

For palaeontologist Stephen Jay Gould (1997) the would-be science of evolutionary psychology, which he refers to disparagingly as a 'superficially attractive cult', only relies on *post hoc* theoretical suppositions and spurious empirical evidence. The history of human development is far too convoluted and the available data far too imprecise and scanty to make definite statements linking how humans presently think, behave, and feel the way they do with what happened over hundreds of thousands of years (Scull, 2007b).

Furthermore, madness has become medicalised and the mad considered in the main maladapted rather than adaptive by psychiatry. Therefore, is psychiatry itself not an adaptive institution but societally maladaptive? That is, if psychiatry (except for its few 'evolutionary' practitioners) is not recognising the personal and cultural purposefulness of what it brands as depression, anxiety, schizophrenia and psychopathy, then rather than helping individuals and being socially useful is it not hindering genetic and memetic evolution?

Raymond Tallis

Raymond Tallis (1946–), neuroscientist, philosopher, humanist and previously a Professor of Geriatric Medicine at the University of Manchester, questions the legitimacy of both evolutionary psychology and neuropsychiatry. For him the scientific claims of these approaches which ultimately reduce human performance to biology are nonsense. When neuroscience and Darwinism trespass into the study of humans and their cultures, Tallis (2011) argues, they evolve into 'neuromania' and 'Darwinitis'. That is, these ideas become mantras rather than well worked-out theories aligned with well-researched evidence and as such are misleading if not dangerous because of the reductionist implications regarding treatment.

Tallis contributes an insightful observation to support his condemnation of how the concepts and data from neuroscience and evolutionary psychology are massively overplayed when applied to psychological states. What Tallis points out is that how the person being studied experiences and interprets his/her feelings, thoughts and behaviours, together with what is seen, heard, smelled and tasted, does not necessarily correspond to the conjectures of the neuroscientist and the evolutionary psychologist. Moreover, what is inferred by those analysing the pictures from imaging scans and information from nucleic acid sequencing, as well as what is invoked by those gazing back into the murky depths of human history and pre-history, is not necessarily the same as what is actually happening within the biology of humans (or any other life-form) or did occur in humanity's past. There is an unavoidable disjunction, big or small, between reality (if there is a reality in the first place) and the ideas which purport to represent that reality. This disjunction is not so surprising because collecting all relevant material about any material event in order to know that event thoroughly is probably impossible. However, to have a science or sciences founded on flaky knowledge which could have such dramatic impact on vulnerable subjects – altering an individual's genes, brain anatomy or bio-chemistry – is once again a vital ethical issue.

As Scull submits (2011), biological reductionism (and its corollary biological determinism) is attractive as an explanation for the families of the mad because they have the opportunity to absolve themselves of any blame for their relatives' condition. Such blame has been laid on relatives by those who embrace the ideas of Laing and before him Bateson (see Chapters 2 and 3). Seeking aberration in the configuration of the brain, imbalances in neurochemicals and neurotransmitters, and defective genes, argues Scull, is more acceptable to relatives in terms of accountability than having a (renegade) psychiatrist seemingly uncovering double-binds and scapegoating in family life. But, this is not a logical argument put forward by Scull. Families, especially parents, may become just as worried about attracting blame for their faulty biology which they share with and may have passed on to their offspring as they would be for imperfect interpersonal relationships.

Teleology tenuousness

As is pointed out by Tallis, providing evidence to connect specific neurological abnormalities with specific mental abnormalities is definitely complex and probably misconceived. Only rarely may precise and confident cause-and-effect relationships be indicated. Moreover, Tallis is implying that in many instances neuroscientists are using the specious argumentative style of teleology. Teleology means listing the characteristics of a phenomenon to define what it is, and then explaining what it is by listing its characteristics. Brain pathologies are being 'described' as particular mental disorders and *vice versa* and not 'explained'. Diagnostic description rather than explanation was apparent in the case of Cahalan, not only between but within a number of medical specialities – including neurology.

Moreover, the description may be compiled through the censual outcome of discussions by those seeking a definition, the judgements of one or more 'experts', or a wider caucus encompassing lay opinions. These techniques are inherently arbitrary and subjective, offering compromised or exclusive depictions, not objective enlightenment. Psychiatry is accused of using this circular and insufficient mode of argument to justify the existence of many if not most mental disorders (Bentall, 2009; Read and Dillon, 2013).

Allen Frances, the chair-person of the task force which produced the DSM-IV in 1994, has spoken publically and vociferously against the catch-all category of 'somatic symptom disorder', a diagnosable mental disorder when physical symptoms are reported by the patient but no physical cause can be found:

> [The] DSM 5 has failed us … DSM 5 has decided to proceed on its mindless and irresponsible course. The sad result will be the mislabeling of potentially millions of people with a fake mental disorder [specifically, 'somatic symptom disorder'] that is unsupported by science and flies in the face of common sense.
>
> *Frances, 2013b*

Frances goes on to accuse the American Psychiatric Association of being incompetent because of its failure to supply a diagnostic system which is scientifically robust and thereby, will detrimentally affect many individuals and their families who are given an unsafe diagnosis. The title of his book in which he explains in detail his critical position, not just regarding the DSM but the whole psychiatric enterprise provides a crisp summary of his stance: *Saving Normal: An Insider's Revolt Against Out-Of-Control Psychiatric Diagnosis, Dsm-5, Big Pharma, and the Medicalization of Ordinary Life* (Frances, 2014).

Moreover, the making of mental disorder by a self-selecting few reaching a consensus or perhaps compromise can be reversed. The doyens of psychiatric diagnosis can remove as well as compose mental disorder, and in so doing exercise their power to adjust what part of human performance succumbs to medicalisation and which to de-medicalisation (Greenberg, 2014). Homosexuality and masturbatory-insanity have disappeared from psychiatry's listings of mental disorders. The same fate has happened to narcissistic personality disorder which in the DSM-IV has been relegated to the category of symptom of other personality disorders. Again, however, criticism of this move came from within psychiatry with John Gunderson, a medical specialist in personality disorders, denouncing the sub-committee dealing with that category as 'unenlightened' (Gunderson quoted in Zanor, 2010). In the alternative classification to the DSM, the World Health Organisation's International Classification of Diseases, narcissistic personality disorder was recorded only in an appendix for mental disorders in its tenth version formulated in the early 1990s, but it appears under the heading 'other specific personality disorders' in the 2010 revised version (World Health Organisation, 2010).

Philosopher Peter Hacker focuses on yet another elementary lapse in logic when activities in the brain are not attributed to interactions with other biological systems and departments of the mind or to the whole person. Moreover, for Hacker the absence of accounting for interactions of society and the whole person, including his/her brain, is a further illogicality. These miscarriages of reasoning for Hacker result in:

> [A] false confidence that the natural sciences can explain such historical and cultural facts as why Hannibal did not attack Rome after the battle of Cannae or why Raphael painted Democritus with boots on.
>
> *Hacker in Robinson and Williams, 2015, p.98*

Burying and torturing

Journalist Robert Whitaker, and Lisa Cosgrove (2015), Professor of Counselling at the University of Massachusetts Boston, argue that the corrupting influence of the pharmaceutical industry and the bias and financial interests of the American Psychiatric Association are paramount in what becomes accepted and acceptable knowledge by psychiatry especially in the USA. For them, biological research is erroneously endorsed as providing solid support for intervening in the biology of the individual which may in the first place be erroneously diagnosed.

Negative results from such research are 'buried' and data which may have only a small degree of positivity is 'tortured' until its importance appears to stand out. The psychiatric discourse is dominated by vested commercial interests which push particularly profitable products in the direction of the patient. The propagandising and propagating of drugs and the pathologising of normality lead to serious side effects which may be worse than the predicament for which the person is being treated. Human rights are transgressed regularly, for example, because consent to treatment is not sought or if sought then the implications are not suitably clarified. Whilst most psychiatrists are well-meaning, the institution of psychiatry has failed on nearly all of its undertakings with regard to evidence and efficacy (Whitaker and Cosgrove, 2015).

A future epistemological format for psychiatry based largely on neuroscience would also lessen the need to 'hear' patients, although what they say would still need to be heeded but only to affirm a pre-set diagnosis or to infer the existence of a novel disorder. Psychiatry allied to neurology would allow the power of this amalgamated sub-set of the medical profession to blossom and herald a new age of medical dominance over the mad. However, the implication of Szasz's thesis and that of Cahalan's experience is that psychiatry should be replaced by rather than empowered by neurology.

Oliver James

Oliver James (1953–) is psychodynamic psychologist who also has a background in social anthropology. He has authored articles and texts and has been engaged with various media productions most of which is in the domain of popularised psychology. His 'selfish capitalism' treatise is mentioned in Chapter 4.

James has entered the field of genetics, publishing a book titled *Not In Your Genes: The Real Reasons Children Are Like Their Parents* (James, 2016) in which he attacks the idea that with human performance nature overrides nurture and in particular the way evidence from the Human Genome Project is used to condone biological determinism. James condemns Richard Dawkins for portraying humans as 'mere carcasses' for the transmission of DNA from one generation to another. Humans are not simply conduits for selfish genes but multi-dimensional, interactive, cognate and reflexive forms of life which cannot be reduced to the elemental parts of their complex sum.

There is convincing empirical evidence of harmful genetic mutations causing physical conditions such as cystic fibrosis and muscular dystrophy. There is also declaration by genetic scientists that the genetic complexities of an increasing number of cancers, heart diseases and mental disorders, will be unravelled. Such knowledge evokes the promise of new pharmaceutical interventions to amend genetic malformations and the prospect of altering the future of humanity through the precipitative engineering, slicing, and editing of genes (Megget, 2016; Mukherjee, 2016).

However, James is adamant that none of the extant studies have proven that either unitary genes or a combination of genes affect significantly how intelligence, personality, or psychological distress which come to be diagnosed as mental disorder and treated as though it was caused by biological deficits. Moreover, he argues that there have been enough studies produced on genetics to be able to conclude that no such fundamental and prodigious cause-and-effect relationships will ever be found for most if not all elements of human performance.

Despite regular declarations of genetic discoveries, incontrovertible evidence pointing to a specific genetic cause for most let alone all incidents of manic-depression or schizophrenia is yet to be found (Deacon, 2013). Moreover, in general, it is not one gene that is being hunted by geneticists but an intricate matrix of genes which could have convoluted relationships with multiple neurochemicals. Evidence of anatomical abnormities which may or may not be related to the responsible genetic-neurochemical-bundle may further thwart the search.

Furthermore, speculation continues about other aspects of physiology to those originating involving directly the nerves or chemicals of the brain. For example, inter-systemic immune reactions or inaction may have to be added to the potpourri of biological risk factors (Purcell, *et al.*, 2009; Yang, 2011; Psychiatric Genomics Consortium, 2014; Kerner, 2014).). Complexity, therefore, abounds in the 'biological pathways' along which neurological abnormalities travel to their destination of mental disorder with novel routes appearing regularly (Psychiatric Genomics Consortium, 2015). There are also the confounding factors of people diagnosed with a mental disorder who do not have the supposed genetic/neurological fault and those who are not so diagnosed who do (Connor, 2015).

Childhood and cortisol

All of these biological gradations and provisos are aside from those originating purely in the nuanced spheres of the psyche and the social. Somewhat surprisingly for a clinical psychologist, James seems to forget about the discrete workings of the 'mind' in his categorical exclamation about what he regards as primary in the moulding of human performance and the making of madness:

> The Environment, Stupid!
>
> *James, 2016, p.5*

The most important environmental influence and the most important time to be influenced by the environment for James is the family and childhood. There is, James contends, copious substantive evidence to show that abuse in childhood is a major source of psychological difficulties in later life. There is recognition by James of the part that biology plays when a child is abused. Traumatic situations in early life lead to bio-chemical reactions which in themselves can furnish physical harm. Specifically, the hormone cortisol, which is key to the operation of 'flight or fight' when confronted by threats may be overproduced and/or produced continuously no matter that the perceived danger may be imagined or minimal. Cortisol in this mode can cause anxiety, depression, damage the circulatory system and shorten life. This is not a genetic issue, points out James, but an effect of the social milieu which instigates a biological effect.

Moreover, James dismisses what he refers to as the 'bit of both' approach to understanding human performance and madness. Nurturing and kindly handling on the one hand or neglectful and cruel happenings, especially in childhood, surpass any inherited factor. What is also dismissed by James is the notion of epigenetics. Epigenetics is an unsettled field of study but one which attends to the idea that the environment may impinge on genes at the level of the phenotype. That is, it is not the arrangement of DNA which is affected. It is how the environment operates to switch on and off the presentational aspects of the individual's genetic constitution (Moore, 2015). What James argues is that the unsurmountable difficulty in epigenetic theorising concerns heritability. Research into epigenetics has not and cannot fulfil the gap in the contention from those who regard nature as dictating, for example, that those with tribulations of the mind have inherited these from their parents, or other blood-relatives.

James, based on his evaluation of evidence from studies into genetics and from the sequencing of the human genome, and the validity of conclusions for that research and sequencing, sums up his position thus: genes do not explain why some people are rich and others are poor; genes do not explain social success; genes do not explain madness. With regard to the latter, he provides the example of research into schizophrenia which he contends indicates a close link between sexual abuse in childhood and the later occurrence of the condition. He also mentions the research into schizophrenia that points to emotional abuse, especially over-controlling parenting.

Blaming parents for schizophrenia is an idea which Laing (see Chapter 3) promulgated, and James does imply in this book an admiration at least for Laing's somewhat opaque aphorisms with direct quotes such as 'we are the veils that veil us from ourselves' (Laing quotes in James, 2016, p.58) this one about families:

> We are acting parts in a play we have never read or never seen, whose plot we don't know, whose existence we can glimpse but whose beginning and end are beyond our imagination and conception.
>
> *Laing quoted in James, 2016, p.111*

But what James offers is a caricature of genetic research and researchers. It cannot be predicted, indeed it is not good science to state resolutely, that genes (or by implication non-genetically triggered neurological malfunction) will never be found to cause madness. Although James is disparaging of the 'bit of both' position, most geneticists do accept the role of the environment in how humans perform. It is not either/or, it is biological, psychological and social. For example, neuroscientist McGuffin (in Rose and McGuffin, 2005) accepts explicitly that biology interplays with psycho-social factors. Psychiatrist and neuroscientist Bruce Wexler (2006) appreciates that the social environment affects the structure and functioning of the brain. That is, the plasticity of brain matter allows it to adjust to social stimuli.

Another straw-man

Hence, what James is expounding is another 'straw-man' argument. The 'straw-man' accusation, and many other accusations is made by psychology researcher Stuart Ritchie who has delivered a hard-hitting attack review of James's book. Ritchie describes James' foray into genetics as:

> a compendium of psychological myths and legends.
>
> *Ritchie, 2016*

It is preposterous, argues Ritchie, for James to declare repeatedly that because so far only a small number of genes have been allied to particular traits such as schizophrenia, that genetic causation can be dismissed. What is more logical and scientific, suggests Ritchie, is to accept that such connections may be discovered. Ritchie accuses James of a high level of intellectual naïveté concerning the robustness, implications and potential of genetic research. Such cerebral constraint, implies Ritchie, is not apparent amongst geneticists given that the majority of these would recognise that the environment plays its part in how humans perform, a proposition James disdains, as well as appreciating the present nascent state of their research.

In part, Ritchie continues, James's scholarly limitations are to be expected because of him existing in a 'neo-Freudian world'. What Ritchie seems to be inferring is that James is preconditioned to view the work of geneticists through the prism of Freudian concepts and thereby is not susceptible to accepting that there may be some legitimacy to their approach and findings. However, this denunciation can be levelled at all of those embedded in specialisms, including Ritchie.

But Ritchie extends his condemnation of James to include all of his popular publications. For Ritchie much damage to the public's understanding of science, the human psyche and schizophrenia has been done because of James's 'scientific illiteracy' and 'mediocre writing' and appearances in the media which are often 'shriekingly aggressive'. What Ritchie calls for is a 'realistic' view of these subjects.

W L

If the input of genetic-neurological ideas into psychiatry is based at worst on unsubstantiated empiricism, misguided logic, institutionalised corruption, and inappropriate conflation of normality with madness, and at best on exaggerated or embryonic accomplishment and predictions, then how secure is Cahalan's diagnosis or any other past or present category of psychiatry?

General paralysis of the insane

The uncounted numbers of people who came to be described as suffering from 'general paralysis of the insane'[4] serve as a reminder of psychiatry's success in finding the cause of a fatal madness and eventually a cure. Moreover, it was and continues to be drawn upon to exemplify the scientific status and biological basis of psychiatry. However, general paralysis of the insane also serves as an example of interpretative ephemerality and variability in psychiatric classifications and paradigms. Even the name changes depending on the epoch and the interests of those who are expounding on the condition. Over the centuries since it was suspected to be a specific condition, it has been given many appellations apart from general paralysis of the insane, for example, general paralysis, dementia paralytica, tertiary syphilis, neuro-syphilis and Bayle's Disease.

General paralysis of the insane had been regarded as a specific condition by British surgeon and apothecary at Bethlem/Bedlam John Haslam (1798) at the end of the eighteenth century and again in the 1820s by French physical Antoine Bayle. Bayle invigorated Haslam's limited portrayal and trumped the eminent Esquirol's (1845) formulation. He, unlike his professional superior, understood that insanity was the effect not the cause of a disorder suffered by nearly a third of the patients entering Charenton Hospital in Paris where he had gone to work in 1818. Bayle's irregular idea, which he presented in his PhD thesis using his observation of post-mortem examination of six affected brains, was that this form of madness stemmed from some factor outside of the brain (Kaplan, 2010). His description of the inflammation and destruction of tissue in the brain and his pointing to external causation was pioneering and for psychiatry's scientific aspirations it is exemplary:

> [Bayle's discovery] deserves to go down in history as the *fons et orgigo* of the scientific roots of the discipline.
>
> *Kaplan, 2010, p.19*

There are disputes about the actual origin of syphilis but the most frequently cited source for its appearance in Europe is attributed to the disarrayed French armies of Charles VIII in the late sixteenth century which deposited an assortment of infectious and disabling diseases as they retreated from Italy and headed back to their own country. But syphilis may have been brought to Europe by the early Spanish explorers returning from the Americas (Franzen, 2008).

Arsenic and mercury

It was the zoologist Fritz Schaudin and dermatologist Erich Hoffman, both German, who in 1905 identified the bacteria, Spirochaeta pallida, which was named later Treponema pallidum, as being the responsible agent for syphilis. A year later the first diagnostic test was produced by the German microbiologist and immunologist August von Wasserman. Syphilis was also found to be congenital, passed on from an infected mother to her foetus (Nicol, 1956).

For hundreds of years previously, the condition was treated with mercury. From 1910 several different compounds of arsenic were formulated as treatments. One of these compounds, Salvarsan, was found to be effective and had the benefit of neither producing horrendous side effects nor killing its recipient (Franzen, 2008).

Later that century the deliberate infecting of syphilitic patients with tuberculin or malaria became treatments of choice due to the observation by clinicians that high fever reduced the symptoms of severe madness. 'Fever therapy' had been tried during medieval times for various assumed types of somatic and psychological disturbances. In 1917, whilst the First World War was raging in Europe, Austrian psychiatrist Julius Wagner-Jauregg was to receive on one of his wards which usually only accepted soldiers with considerable psychological difficulties a minor casualty who was also suffering from malaria. What Wagner-Jauregg decided to do was withhold treatment in the form of Quinine from the malarial soldier and to take some of his blood which was then rubbed into the wounds of three of his patients who had also been diagnosed with general paralysis of the insane. The apparent success of this dangerous and ethically questionable experiment was, 10 years later, to earn Wagner-Jauregg a Nobel Prize (Nicol, 1956).

Tuskegee and penicillin

No such accolade was to be awarded to the researchers who conducted what was titled 'Tuskegee Study of Untreated Syphilis in the Negro Male'. The study, which took place in Tuskegee, Alabama in the USA, commenced in 1932 and ran for 40 years. Six hundred male African-Americans, many impoverished and illiterate, were recruited as participants. Two-thirds of these men had been diagnosed with syphilis, with the rest used as a control group (Jones, 1993).

The purpose of the study was to observe how syphilis evolved amongst this section of the population. No participant was told by the researchers that he had syphilis, nor what was the purpose of the study, nor how his health might deteriorate. What they were told was that they had 'bad blood', a parochial phrase which covered a series of diseases. Enticements to participate included free meals and free medical treatment for any minor conditions, and the promise that when they died their families would receive monetary benefits. Some treatment was offered but was hazardous or futile or both. They were not offered effective and safe treatment – penicillin – when it became available decades before the end of the study. By the time study ended, over 100 of the men died directly from syphilis or from its complications. Moreover, unknown numbers of the men's sexual partners and whoever those partners may have had sex with, along with their children, were infected with syphilis (Jones, 1993).

It took nearly 20 years after the discovery of penicillin in 1928 before it was to become the treatment of choice for anyone diagnosed with syphilis let alone the participants of the Tuskegee Study. Penicillin was shown to be very proficient at destroying the syphilitic-causing microorganism, and far less risky than introducing potentially poisonous substances or fighting the 'fire' from one disease with the fever from another. Notwithstanding the perils of resistance to antibiotics, penicillin remains the treatment of choice (National Institute for Health and Care Excellence, 2014). Crucially, from the 1940s onwards it could be prescribed to prevent the onset of its most destructive final upshot, that is general paralysis of the insane.

Insanity anonymised

A host of famous painters, poets, philosophers, and political leaders have had their stories told or at least they have had syphilitic sufferings debated and questioned (for example, Friedrich Nietzsche, Wolfgang Amadeus Mozart, Ludwig van Beethoven, Paul Gauguin, Arthur Schopenhauer, Gustave Flaubert and Vladimir Lenin: Franzen, 2008). But the names of the vast majority of sufferers are not known, and their stories have not been told by them nor by anyone else.

What is available are the medical records which tell of a tiny segment of their lives. The documentation reveals intense psychological distress, complete physical disintegration and untimely death.

Kenneth McLeod was a student in Medical Psychology and Mental Diseases at the University of Edinburgh, Scotland and Assistant Medical Officer of the Durham County Asylum, Sedgefield, England. In 1862 McLeod wrote to Thomas Laycock, Professor of the Practice of Medicine at Edinburgh University, providing him with the details of two patients he had been attending. He apologised to Laycock for not sending details earlier. His lateness, McLeod explains, was due to having been very busy with his 'asylum engagements'. These patients, McLeod explains to Laycock, were illustrative of two distinct forms of mania as a consequence of general paralysis of the insane. One of these cases, a man referred to only as 'WL' by McLeod, had a fondness for alcohol. Alongside the nervous system and the 'reflexive' interplay of consciousness and unconsciousness sited in the brain, drunkenness was a focus of Laycock's academic and clinical interest. McLeod's communication to Laycock is recorded in what was then the *Journal of Mental Science*, later retitled as the *British Journal of Psychiatry*.

No one in WL's family, according to McLeod, suffered from madness. Although McLeod doesn't specify where WL spent his childhood, the implication is it was in Northumberland given that his father was a farmer in the locale. However, he worked in his early adult years in Wales as a miner. The personal details of his health, physique and personality are elucidated by McLeod but the source for this information is not explicit. Seemingly WL was as a young man muscular, ruddy complexion, energetic, hard-working and intellectually unimpressive but of a steady, hard-working, sociable, kindly disposition with no indication of eccentricity.

As he grew older, McLeod's history-taking continues, WL became more dissolute. His sexual appetite became driven, and his intake of alcohol increased to a level of habitual inebriation. At this point, WL, according to McLeod, contracted syphilis for which he sought the help of a 'quack'. This quack, writes McLeod, administered copious potions amongst which was mercury but which were injurious rather than effective.

WL in 1855 moved to Newcastle in northern England where he worked as a stone-quarrier, wages from which were very generous. He spent most of his money on alcohol, alternating between diligence in his job and intemperance in his social life. His excess alcohol consumption was to affect his personality and led to inappropriate belligerence, occasional episodes of violence, other forms of irrationality. McLeod notes that in the following year, WL apparently had an apoplectic incident, falling into unconsciousness for about an hour, and after which he was slightly paralysed down the right side of his body.

The aftermath of his apoplexy, according to McLeod, involved further degeneration of the intellect and emotional excitability resulting in his admission to Bath Lane Asylum, Newcastle during 1857. On examination at the asylum he was found to be unable to walk or speak properly, to have tremors in his limbs, and to be often extremely irritable but otherwise lethargic. He became fixated on collecting items of any sort, sometimes stealing them from other patients, and hoarding them where ever he could. His urethra showed a discharge and he had two–three small sores on his penis.

The year after admission to Bath Lane Asylum all of the patients were transferred to another nearby institution, Durham County Asylum at Sedgefield. Here, WL was to stay for a further year during which time, McLeod states, he was treated with 'antisyphilitics, astringents, tonics, stimulants, and a generous diet' (McLeod, 1862, p.549) although there is no mention of the precise make-up of these medications. WL's physical deportment and psychological manner fluctuated wildly in the ensuing months but eventually stabilised so that after a few weeks 'trial' in the outside world he was discharged.

WL was brought back to Durham County Asylum in April of 1859. Before re-admission, he had become once again dependent on alcohol, and more violent with occurrences of impulsivity one of which was to order a 'large hot-house for a small garden' (McLeod, 1862, p.551). McLeod recalls that the medical examination of WL this time reveals that his pupils contracted dissimilarly although this was only 'slight'. A difference in the reaction of pupils is indicative of general paralysis of the insane (Pearce, 2004).

Moreover, his attention and memory were poor, his overall physical movements and control were once again uncertain with periods of paralysis, he had much difficulty in speaking, and was lacking in energy except for bouts of fanatical accumulation. Referring to WL's expression, McLeod explains that the clinical transcriptions indicate that it was mostly, emotionless, but could be doleful, tearful and assume a look of 'pain and suffering'. At the age of 39, WL was somatically and psychologically in steep decline.

When McLeod saw WL for the first time early in August of 1861 he was incapable of movement, covered in large pustules and bed-sores which were becoming gangrenous, and 'mentally demented'. Within two weeks WL died.

McLeod performed a post-mortem examination. He lists the intricate details of the condition of the brain. There was obvious pathology in WL's brain coverings (the meninges) although less so in its deeper substance. However, separating normal from abnormal and how the latter may have related to the patient's presenting symptomatology and death, McLeod is unsure, which is why he asked for advice from Laycock. However, there is no suggestion that he doubts WL had contracted syphilis and this had resulted in his death from the effects of general paralysis of the insane.

Heroic respectability

Had penicillin been available to prescribe to WL then he may have lived into old age. Once penicillin became available for prescription, syphilis could be stopped well before it reached its tertiary stage. Eventually, the asylums would not be replete with those who had reached that stage (Davis, 2012).

So, psychiatry can be successful. However, as noted by Juliet Hurn (1998) in her ground-breaking thesis on the history of general paralysis of the insane, this indisputable but isolated success has led to an overconfidence and blinkered positioning of psychiatry not only as a science but as a biological science. Hurn does not reject the biology of general paralysis of the insane but considers its cultural meanings and in particular its role in fostering the social advance of psychiatry.

General paralysis of the insane, Hurn comments, has been for psychiatry a matchless scientific model attuned to biology but the history of the disorder and that of its place in promoting this medical subdivision as a science is only one of many historical accounts which could be presented. The social and physical environment in which both the disorder and medical subdivision arose and proliferated need to be viewed as contributing profoundly to what was to become the prevailing history of psychiatry. That is, the one that highlighted the heroism of psychiatrists in finding coherent categories of disorder, causes, and cures for all of madness and the hope of psychiatry that it would become a respectable branch of the medicine profession.

However, had the venereologists been more occupationally ambitious, or post-mortem practices and laboratory technology not either been accommodated by those medical practitioners with an interest in the association biology – especially the brain – has with madness, had not these practitioners been willing to expose their patients to the perils of experimental remedies, had the Spanish sailors not returned home and/or French soldiers stayed at home, had nineteenth century men been less sexually profligate and prostitutes fewer, then the history of syphilis and psychiatry might be very different.

Hurn also mentions the remarks made by Szasz (1976b) about syphilis and psychiatry. For Szasz, the medicalisation of madness on the back of psychiatry's success with one disorder is a 'scientific scandal'. The characteristics and consequences of that achievement have been inappropriately extended to cover most, if not all, forms of madness without, Szasz argues, any scientific justification.

Nikolas Rose

But, rather than division can there be a paradigm, possibly a revolutionary one, which synthesises social science and psychiatric science, which amalgamates and improves the knowledge of both for the benefit of those people who may be or have been voted mad? Nikolas Rose along with Joelle Abi-Rached, a PhD student in the history of science at Harvard University, calls for such a paradigmatic shift.

Rose (1947–) first trained as a biologist then took an interest in psychology before embarking on a long and distinguished career in sociology. He has written about a multitude of social scientific subjects (Rose, 2016). These comprise: the organisation, systems, and effects of psychology and other 'psye' disciplines on the self and society; the social history of the social sciences, law and crime; political power and the different ways governments advance their legitimacy; creeds and formations of risk; how subjectivity and 'the soul' is fashioned and experienced; and consumers and consumption. He has also been writing about psychiatry and madness for decades and is the co-author of a seminal text on these topics, *The Power of Psychiatry* (Miller and Rose, 1986), which I have referred to elsewhere in this book. Latterly, Rose (2010; 2013) has turned his academic attention to social scientific critique of biology. Rose has narrowed his scrutiny of biology to examine neuroscience.

Neuromolecular gaze

Rose and Abi-Rached argue that there was an epistemological move beginning in the 1960s which they term 'the neuromolecular gaze'. This new positioning in the study of human biology is exceptionally reductionist as it moves scientific and psychiatric technology and thinking into looking at and conceptualising the most minuscule of workings in the body and especially the brain (Abi-Rached and Rose, 2010; Rose and Abi-Rached, 2013). However, rather than indulging in mere criticism of this development, although they do offer much censorship, Rose and Abi-Rached propose a synthesising of ideas generated by social science and neuroscience. A productive engagement between the social sciences and neuroscience, they argue, could benefit both disciplines.

Rose and Abi-Rached explore the meaning of the neuromolecular gaze for society and individuals, and ponder what exactly shapes human performance, whether that be classified as normal or abnormal. They reject what they refer to as the 'simplifications' of sociobiology and evolutionary psychology and the equally simplistic phrase espoused by purists of biological determinism that 'mind is what brain does' (Rose and Abi-Rached, 2013, p.3). Human performances such as falling in love, empathy, hostility, a fixation on material possessions, deviancy and madness, cannot be summoned-up by mapping out and postulating on the intricacies of DNA, synapses and compounds. They also rehearse the 'biopolitical' corollaries of focusing on biology to account for human performance. Issues of social power and individual freedom are affected by how much society, and behaviour, emotions, and feelings and madness are projected as being orchestrated by biology.

They trace a surge in psychiatry's commitment to having its knowledge and practices re-positioned to be based on genetics and neuroscience back to the beginning of the twentieth century and observe that this has now swelled into a prized policy by the major psychiatric research institutions. This is not least because psychiatry's attention to genetics and neuroscience attracts large-scale funding and gives scientific credibility, and this is not least due to the interest of those commercial industries with products to sell on the back of genetic and neuroscientific research.

As James has commented, however, all of the funding, technologies, and studies have not in the main linked specific biomarkers to specific disorders:

> Despite the penetrating gaze of neuroscience … psychiatric classification remains superficial. This neuromolecular vision seems incapable of grounding the clinical work of psychiatry in a way that has become routine in other areas of medicine.
>
> *Rose and Abi-Rached, 2013, p.138*

For Rose and Abi-Rached madness is not a problem to be understood in the laboratory but of the individual in his/her society's culture and history. Furthermore, neuroscience and psychiatry have also to be placed in time and space. They are social institutions staffed by social beings.

But, unlike what is implied by James, they do not accuse most of the promoters of the neuromolecular gaze of deterministic purity. They acknowledge that the ontology of humans is not formulated by the majority of today's neuroscientists as purely dictated by genes, brain mechanisms, and chemicals in the brain or affecting the brain but originating elsewhere in the body. Neuroscientists have grasped that the brain is 'plastic', a reflexive organ. Nature and nurture interact and in doing so each can alter (Eagleman, 2016). However, Rose and Abi-Rached, point out that the biopolitical sequelae of accepting the occurrence of neuro-plasticity is an increase in the 'new-liberal' obligation for individuals to take increased responsibility for their own self. If humans have the ability to modify their social as well as their physical environment and are not just irresolute brains, bio-chemistry, and sequences of DNA, then they can be blamed for their own deviancies including those concerning their psychological states and the State can opt out of its duties and put aside charges of incompetence or malevolence.

Bio-psycho-social brain

However, Rose and Abi-Rached submit that no matter how unlikely, neuroscience can be an ally of progressive social thinking and societal change. It is the recognition by neuroscience that the brain is not only biological but 'social', that it exerts influence on and is influenced by society, that provides the opening for social scientists and scientists (and psychiatrists) to work on improving the lot of people and their surroundings.

Neuroscientists Christopher Butler and Adam Zeman (2015) point out that many neurological disorders may be mistaken for psychiatric ones, although the reverse can also occur. For example, certain forms of dementia may not only present with major changes in speech and gait but alter personality dramatically. A physical (neurological) disorder, therefore, may be considered as psychological and dealt with accordingly but erroneously. Butler and Zeman argue rather than rescuing patients from mistaken notions and specious settings, and because physical and psychological symptoms are interlinked, then whatever the setting, a bio-psycho-social model of diagnosis and treatment should be adopted.

The synthesis of social science and scientific psychiatry has also been recommended by medical practitioners and much earlier than Rose. One notable such protagonist is child psychiatrist and social psychiatrist Leon Eisenberg. Eisenberg advocated the coming together of sociological and psychiatric ideas. He remarked as far back as the 1970s that both physical and psychological disorders reflect interaction which involves the structure and content of both biology and society no matter what is their frank triggers, presentation and remedies (Eisenberg, 1977). For example, smoking cigarettes and the occurrence of lung cancer concerns toxins, neoplastic growths, radiotherapy, surgery and chemotherapy, as well as that of advertising, cooperate clout, education, public opinion and government policies relating to taxation and availability.

Eisenberg and the psychiatrist and anthropologist Arthur Kleinman, whose work is discussed in Chapter 4, proposed decades ago that brain structure is moulded by social experience (Eisenberg and Kleinman, 1980). For them, sociology and anthropology need to be conjoined with the science of biology in dealing with the prevention and curing of ill-health. They challenged medical practitioners and social scientists to work with each other:

> Just as physicians need an appreciation of what social science can contribute to the understanding of patienthood [sic] and healing ... social scientists must immerse themselves in the clinic in order to relate theory to practice with a better appreciation of the urgencies and immediacies of patient care.
>
> *Eisenberg and Kleinman, 1980, p.19*

More recently, Simon Wessely psychiatrist and Professor of Psychological Medicine at the Institute of Psychiatry, King's College London, has argued for a 'holistic' approach. For him, psychiatry is the study of the brain and the mind. As such, what is needed is the application of biology, sociology and psychology along with many other social scientific subjects to understand their interconnectedness. Significantly, he suggests that psychiatrists and biologists have become tired of the hackneyed debate which separates nature from nurture.

It is both he claims (Wessely, quoted in Wessely and James, 2013). The job of the psychiatrist, he argues, is to look after the whole of the person.

There is an academic and clinical speciality tagged 'social neuroscience' (Cacioppo and Berntson, 1992; Todorov *et al.*, 2014). Its nomenclature signifies the synthesis of nurture and nature regarding human performance. The neuroscientist David Eagleman (2016) is a protagonist of 'social neuroscience' and reports that humans are 'social creatures' and accepts that nature and nurture affect each.

A conference in 2015 was held by the British Royal Society of Medicine in London under the banner of 'Psychiatry and society: will neuroscience change understandings and practices?'. Together with distinguished neuroscientists, social scientist Nikolas Rose was one of the speakers and David Armstrong, Professor of Medicine and Sociology, King's College London was on the discussion panel at the end of the conference. Aims of the conference included the exploration of the impact of genetics and neuroscience on understandings of mental disorder, and the promotion of dialogue between psychiatrists, biomedical scientists and social scientists (Royal Society of Medicine, 2015).

There is willingness from within psychiatry and social science to share their knowledge with a view to furnishing more thorough understandings of present positions and potentially creating novel conceptions of and practices affecting madness. However, how much of this is ineffectual tokenism (unintended presumably) versus a substantive movement remains to be seen.

Some professions which deal with people diagnosed as mentally disordered have been receptive possibly since their inception, to the notion that society matters. Social work traditionally and markedly has been one of these professions, but there are moves to disengage from a simplistic causative binary divide which separates faults within individual from faults in society (Karban, 2011). The medical profession is also not unreceptive to a nuanced view of causation which accepts the interplay of biological and social conditions for some mental disorders and the latter being the root of a few others (National Library of Medicine, 2016). Moreover, even where biological markers have been thought to be identified, for example, for schizophrenia and manic-depression (Cross-Disorder Group of the Psychiatric Genomics Consortium, 2013), there is caution from medical researchers about the degree to which these indicate a risk of mental disorder (National Institutes of Health, 2013). Research into epigenetics, that is the ways in which genes are altered by an individual's experiences in social and physical environments, is one nuanced approach (Weir, 2012).

Shrinks and pluralism

Jeffrey Lieberman is a modern psychiatrist with impeccable scientific qualifications. He is Chairman of Psychiatry at Columbia University's College of Physicians and Surgeons, and Psychiatrist in Chief at Columbia University Medical Centre-New York Presbyterian Hospital, and Director of the New York

State Psychiatric Institute. Lieberman is also a former President of the American Psychiatric Association who was responsible for overseeing the drawing-together and implementation in 2013 of the DSM-V. In his book, written with computational neuroscientist Ogi Ogas and published in 2015, *Shrinks: The Untold Story of Psychiatry*, he repackages the positive chronicling of his profession which had originally been set-out by medical historian Edward Shorter (1997: see Chapter 2).

What Lieberman does in *Shrinks* is to praise the scientific achievements of psychiatry and in particular the purpose and veracity of the DSM-V. However, he is not unswervingly rapturous about biology being the only basis on which the epistemological edifice of his profession should rest, and nor is he unwaveringly persuaded on that idea's concomitant methods of treatment. Research into genetics and the invention of a plethora of scans to uncover the malfunctioning of the brain, alongside improvements in the efficacy of psycho-pharmaceuticals, have enormously enhanced the scientific status of psychiatry, or rather for Lieberman they should have so done. However, at a time when Lieberman believes psychiatry is rebirthing as a worthy division of the medical profession because of, in his view, its remarkable advances, he wants to gestate pluralism.

There are, argues Lieberman, psychotherapies which demonstrated their credibility scientifically, such as cognitive-behavioural-therapy which therefore can be included in the arsenal of remedies available for psychiatry to dispense. Indeed, cognitive-behavioural-therapy, along with similar 'evidence-based' psychotherapies, is thriving largely because it calls upon science to sanction its integrity (Layard and Clark, 2014). Moreover, he does make mention of social elements regarding the causation of madness including poverty, racism and disharmonious family relationships as well as undefined 'psycho-social' interventions.

What Lieberman does not do is to offer much if any detail about social causation, sociologically informed therapies or the readjustment of society as a method of moderating madness. Moreover, his 'story of psychiatry' is one which is embedded in the USA and pays scant attention to cultural variation internal or external to that country. Furthermore, he not only attacks anti-psychiatrists some of whose actions he claims have been detrimental to their patients, and Sigmund Freud for leading scientific psychiatry into an 'intellectual desert' for more than 50 years, but he also criticises social scientists such as Erving Goffman and David Rosenhan (see Chapter 3). Hence, Lieberman is very selective about which alternative ideas can be reared in his pluralist fold.

Lieberman refers to the fifth version of the DSM being a 'living document'. This is signified, he reports, in the changing of the Roman numeral 'V' (this style of numbering being used in previous editions of the DSM) to '5'. This change, he points out, indicates that other versions would be forthcoming.

Such fiddling with the DSM, however, may also indicate that mental disorder is an unstable arrangement of aspects of human performance and that ideas about madness beyond his advocated family of scientifically approved perspectives should still be considered.

Summary

Despite what would appear to be an accurate diagnosis eventually having been found for Cahalan's 'month of madness' that does not mean unreservedly that this knowledge is immutable. Arguably, societal conditions affect paradigms of knowledge and thereby how conditions of human performance are concocted and handled.

A future history of madness may recall how Cahalan's madness rather than being Dalmar's Disease may have been a different neurological disorder, or not a neurological disorder but another type of physical or mental disorder, or possibly a state of being classifiable using a paradigm of thought yet to be invented. After all, hysteria as a specific mental disorder is no longer included in psychiatry's formal diagnostic lexicons, and its inventor Freud, had turned from his original paradigm of neurology to that of his invention, psychoanalysis. There are different histories that can be told, suggests Hurn, concerning that seemingly most sound exemplar of a neurological disorder, one which fomented the biological model of madness, general paralysis of the insane.

The projected normalising of neuroscience and genetics as the dominant science(s) psychiatry could become disparaged just as earlier ideas and practices became ridiculed from within and outside psychiatry – mass incarceration and ice-picks come to mind. The revolution may start anytime.

Notes

1 The distinction between neurology and neuroscience is habitually blurred in the clinical literature. However, the tendency is to consider the former as a medical speciality which is supported by the concepts and data arising from the latter. Moreover, neuroscience embraces many practices and practitioners other than those with a background or interest in neurology (Martin, 2002).
2 Also known as 'psychoimmunology', 'psycho-neuro-immunology', neuro-immunology and psychoneuroimmunology.
3 Stephen Rose and Nikolas Rose, whose work is discussed later in this chapter, are brothers.
4 I have deliberately not, after first use, abbreviated 'general paralysis of the insane' to 'GPI' to avoid diminishing the impact and implications of the full designation.

Further reading

Cahalan, S. (2012) *Brain on Fire: My Month of Madness*. London: Penguin.
James, O. (2016) *Not In Your Genes: The Real Reasons Children are Like Their Parents*. London: Vermillion.
Lieberman, J. (2015) *Shrinks: The Untold Story of Psychiatry*. London: Weidenfeld & Nicolson.
Rose, N. and Abi-Rached, J. (2013) *Neuro: The New Brain Sciences and the Management of the Mind*. Princeton, New Jersey, USA: Princeton University Press.

CONCLUSION

This book began with a quotation from the seventeenth century playwright Nathaniel Lee in which he refers to how 'they' had voted him mad. The stories told in this book of people who have been voted mad or who have voted themselves mad is only one story which could have been told about them and the ideas which purport to comprehend their madness are only one set which could have been chosen. What therefore can be voted about madness? I invite you (the reader) to cast your own vote, that is to decide which if any idea for any madness or madness overall is convincing. The stories and ideas which appear in this book have altered my voting behaviour. That is, in researching for this book I have not so much had a personal 'paradigm shift' but an attack of 'cognitive diffidence', an un-medicalised disordered state in thinking.

Realism

Previously, I voted for an idea not mentioned so far, that of 'realism' (Morrall, 1998; 2009). This is an approach which is also adhered to by health sociologist Anne Rogers and clinical psychologist David Pilgrim in their award-winning text titled *A Sociology of Mental Health and Illness*, presently in its fifth edition (Rogers and Pilgrim, 2014).

Realism comes in various guises, for example 'critical realism', and 'new-left realism', and Rogers and Pilgrim's version of 'social realism'. The version which I adopted attempts a synthesis of two opposing positions regarding the natural, personal, and social worlds in general and health/ill-health (physical and psychological) in particular. That there are real facts and a real existence is the core proposition of the first position. This stance is accepted, in the main, by (natural) science, psychiatry and certain sociological theorists such as the 'structuralists'. The second position regards facts and reality as 'made up'. From this position everything in the social, personal and natural worlds (including health/ill-health) is fabricated, there is no one truth and there is an infinitive number of interpretations of existence and experiences. Social constructionism and postmodernism adopt this stance. Variations of one of these two positions are contained in the ideas educed in previous chapters.

The synthesising of these two positions owes much to the work of philosopher Roy Bhaskar (1975; 2008). Bhaskar argues that reality does exist and so do facts, but finding that reality and establishing facts is problematic. This is because eternally, everything everywhere is clouded by subjective interpretations and cultural connotations. Such overlaying of reality and facts with individual perceptions and opinions, and collective values and practices, camouflages underlying certainties. Establishing 'what is true' is made all the more unlikely, argues Bhaskar, because instruments and processes designed to accesses facts and reality are not only imprecise but themselves affected by a multitude of personal and social factors (as has been discussed in Chapter 5).

Humanity has managed to find ways of travelling into outer space, communicating through the ether, splitting the atom and killing bacteria and viruses, but these actual achievements only scratch the surface of the inconceivably intricate and dynamic character of existence. Furthermore, reality is probably inconceivable for humans as they are restricted by the relatively atavistic configuration of their intellectual and sensory equipment. A further tenet of Bhaskar's realism is that individuals are in a reflexive relationship with the world(s) in which they find themselves. This interconnection, however, creates a further complication in terms of establishing stable truths. Bhaskar uses the term 'intransitive knowledge' to describe invariable reality and facts, and 'transitive knowledge' for the personal estimations and cultural clutter which drape reality and facts. What humans are left with are best guesses at comprehending reality, which is reflected in the embryonic, incomplete, if not contradictory data decanted from scientific and social scientific research.

Madness from this perspective has a reality but that reality is muddied due to the individual's specific biological and psychological characteristics and those of his/her social context. The mud if further congealed because of the mix of social sways arising from governmental, academic and clinical partiality. The 'best guess' of psychiatry is fast becoming biased towards neuroscience and genetics, but for social scientists the psychological and societal are favoured.

Abstention

Surprisingly (to me) no longer am I convinced that realism is the best guess, given that for the Bhaskarian realist no actual answer could ever be conclusive. Apart from the realist's pessimistic proposition that reality probably can never be properly portrayed, the distinction between intransitive and transitive knowledge is tricky. Are, for example, all of the principles, descriptions, laws and formulae of physics, chemistry, biology and mathematics, as similarly and permanently unsettled as the knowledge of psychology and sociology?

All of the ideas presented in this book, including realism, have their strengths but also their weaknesses regarding the understanding of madness. Australian psychiatrist Niall McLaren in his book titled *Humanizing Madness* puts it thus:

> Each idea or theory about madness has shortcomings ... Let me, therefore, risk being hoisted by my own petard by claiming boldly that there is no authentic, valid, reliable, robust overarching idea or theory which explains madness.
>
> *McLaren, 2007, p.96*

McLaren does himself present a petard on which to be hoisted by then proposing an idea, one that attempts to humanise psychiatry. He argues for the tempering of the biological fixation of contemporary psychiatry by returning to the old idea that humans have a mind as well as a brain.

As discussed in Chapter 5, however, this allegation of fixation may be misplaced. There are indications from within psychiatry that the mind may be re-installed as a compelling constituent of human performance which is not just the result of genetic and neurological predisposition. As such, there is a rebirthing of an old idea that there needs to be an integration of ideas from otherwise competing disciplines and paradigms. But, the principal problem with combinational ideas such as realism and any bio-psycho-social blend is that they may be merging the weaknesses not the strengths of each element, or merely conflating otherwise incompatible concepts and thereby fostering incoherent consequential practices.

My best guess as of now is that no idea (or mishmash of ideas) about madness can understand madness because it is un-understandable, or rather it becomes understandable only within the terms of that idea/those ideas. No single idea, nor any combination of ideas, understands or can understand madness beyond the limitations of its own paradigmatic boundaries. Furthermore, as observed by Kuhn (1962) there is a temptation for theorists and empiricists to remain within a paradigm, or to only make moderate modifications, no matter that there is evidence to challenge the supporting idea(s). When madness is construed as 'mental disorder', 'social deviancy', 'neuropathology', a mix of intransitive/transitive knowledge, or whatever, what it was it is no longer. It has become a different entity under the terms of the applied idea and its applicants covert their creativity.

Petard

With the realisation that I along with McLaren might fall into a trap of my own making, I offer a proposal, the fertilising of a very old idea from the sociology of Emile Durkheim (2013; original 1895) and Robert Merton (1949). Their 'functionalist' idea acknowledges the interconnectedness of individuals and society and the service supplied to each other.

Madness may serve a purpose in society. Patently, it helps people and society to separate acceptable from unacceptable human performance, and clearly what is acceptable and unacceptable changes from place to place and time to time. Every society delineates normal from abnormal, and reacts (mostly negatively) to what is perceived by the populace and/or the powerful as erratic, bizarre and intimidating acts, thoughts, and emotions (Hirst and Woolley, 1982; Helman, 2007). It follows that unacceptability is marked inevitably with an indelible stigma in most places and across most times. Stigma, therefore, may serve a purpose[1] (Morrall, 2016). But what might be the real purpose of madness, if indeed there is purpose, I am not at all sure. Moreover, as with all of the preceding ideas, functionalism has faults, not least of which is that it like others is teleological and therefore may describe but not explain (Holmwood, 2005).

So, after four decades of working in, teaching about and researching madness, I have become better informed but less able to make a choice about which idea explains insanity. My vote therefore is floating, but may if forced fall on the idea of functional uncertainty.

Note

1   To suggest that stigma may persist because of its societal functional to society is not to condone prejudice nor to detract from managing madness with compassion.

Further reading

Abrahamson, M. (1978) *Functionalism*. New York: Prentice-Hall.

Bhaskar, R. (2010) (revised edition) *Reclaiming Reality: A Critical Introduction to Contemporary Philosophy*. London: Routledge.

Rogers, A. and Pilgrim, D. (2014) (fifth edition) *A Sociology of Mental Health and Illness*. Maidenhead: Open University Press/McGraw-Hill.

BIBLIOGRAPHY

ABC (2002) *All in Mind: The Legacy of the Lobotomy*. ABC [Radio, Australia], 3rd February. www.abc.net.au/radionational/programs/allinthemind/the-legacy-of-the-lobotomy/3494960. [accessed 5th November, 2015].

Abercrombie, N., Hill, S., and Turner, B. (1994) *Dictionary of Sociology*. London: Penguin.

Abi-Rached, J., and Rose, N. (2010) The Birth of the Neuromolecular Gaze. *History of the Human Sciences*, 23(1), pp. 11–36.

Abrahamson, D. (2012) R. D. Laing and Long-stay Patients: Discrepant Accounts of the Refractory Ward and 'Rumpus Room' at Gartnavel Royal Hospital. In: Itten, T., and Young, C. (2012) (editors) *R D Laing: Fifty Years Since the Divided Self*. Ross-on-Wye: PCCS. Chapter 5, pp. 54–68.

Aftab, A. (2014) Mental Illness vs Brain Disorders: From Szasz to DSM-5. 28th February. www.neurologytimes.com/dsm-5-0/mental-illness-vs-brain-disorders-szasz-dsm-5#sthash.KfS3ExlG.dpuf. [accessed 13th January, 2016].

Aho, K. (2014) *Existentialism: An Introduction*. Cambridge: Polity.

Alford, H. (2015) Is Donald Trump Actually a Narcissist? Therapists Weigh In! *Vanity Fair*, 11th November www.vanityfair.com/news/2015/11/donald-trump-narcissism-therapists. [accessed 1st December, 2016].

Alvise, A. (2013) *Psychiatry, Subjectivity, Community. Franco Basaglia and Biopolitics*. Berne, Switzerland: Peter Lang.

American Psychiatric Association (2013) *Diagnostic and Statistical Manual of Mental Disorders*, Fifth Edition (DSM-V). Arlington, VA: American Psychiatric Association.

Ando, V., Claridge, G., and Clark, K. (2014) Psychotic Traits in Comedians. *British Journal of Psychiatry*, 204(1) http://bjp.rcpsych.org/content/early/2014/01/02/bjp.bp.113.134569.full.pdf+html?sid=a9786822-019f-4f0a-8fa8-59440b75b972. [accessed 19th May, 2014].

Andrade, J. (2008) The Inclusion of Antisocial Behavior in the Construct of Psychopathy: A Review of the Research. *Aggression and Violent Behavior*, 13(4), pp. 328–335.

Andress, D. (2006) (second edition) *The Terror: Civil War in the French Revolution*. Kettering: Abacus.

Andrews, J., Briggs, A., Porter, R., Tucker, P., and Waddington, K. (1997) *The History of Bethlem*. London: Routledge.

Andrews, P., and Thomson, A. (2009) The Bright Side of Being Blue: Depression as an Adaptation for Analyzing Complex Problems. *Psychological Review*, 116(3), pp. 620–654.

Arnold, C. (2008) *Bedlam: London and its Mad*. London: Simon and Schuster.

Asad, T. (1995) (editor) *Anthropology and the Colonial Encounter*. New York: Prometheus.

Babiak, P., and Hare, R. (2006) *Snakes In Suits: When Psychopaths Go To Work*. New York: Harper Collins.

Bakan, J. (2004) *The Corporation: The Pathological Pursuit of Profit and Power*. New York: Free Press.

Bangstad, S. (2014) *Anders Breivik and the Rise of Islamophobia*. London: Zed.

Barber, N. (2016) Does Trump Suffer from Narcissistic Personality Disorder? *Psychology Today*, 10th August. https://www.psychologytoday.com/blog/the-human-beast/201608/does-trump-suffer-narcissistic-personality-disorder. [accessed 1st December, 2016].

Barker, F., Hulme, P., and Iverson, M. (1998) (editors) *Cannibalism and the Colonial World*. Cambridge: Cambridge University Press.

Barker, P., and Buchanan-Barker, P. (2008) Mental Health in an Age of Celebrity: the Courage to Care. *Journal of Medical Ethics* (Medical Humanities), 34, pp. 110–114.

Barker, P., and Buchanan-Barker, P. (2011) The Rise in Bipolar Disorder is a Myth. *Psychminded*. www.psychminded.co.uk/news/news2011/feb11/rise-in-bipolar-disorder-is-a-myth002.html. [accessed 21st May, 2012].

Barnes, M., and Berke, J. (1973) (first published 1971 by MacGibbon and Kee) *Two Accounts of a Journey Through Madness*. Harmondsworth: Penguin.

Barnes, M. (2000) *Finale*. http://www.mary-barnes.co.uk/finale.htm. [accessed 6th February, 2014].

Baron-Cohen, S. (2011) *Zero Degrees of Empathy: A New Theory of Human Cruelty*. London: Allen Lane.

Barton, R. (1959) *Institutional Neurosis*. Bristol: John Wright & Sons.

Baruch, G., and Treacher, A. (1978) *Psychiatry Observed*. London: Routledge and Kegan Paul.

Basaglia, F. (1964) La Distruzione Dell'ospedale Psichiatrico come Luogo di Istituzionalizzazione [The Destruction of the Psychiatric Hospital as a Place of Institutionalisation]. http://www.triestesalutementale.it/letteratura/testi/35distr.htm. [accessed 21st March, 2014].

Bateman, A., and Krawitz, R. (2013) *Borderline Personality Disorder: An Evidence-Based Guide for Generalist Mental Health Professionals*. New York: Oxford University Press.

Bateson, G. (1961) *Perceval's Narrative: A Patient's Account of His Psychosis 1830-1832*. Stanford, CA: Stanford University Press.

Bateson, G. (1962) (editor) *Perceval's Narrative: A Patient's Account of His Psychosis 1830–1832*. London: Hogarth Press.

Bateson, G., Jackson, D., Haley, J., and Weakland, J. (1956) Toward a Theory of Schizophrenia. *Behavioral Science*, 1(4), pp. 251–264.

Battye, W. (1758) *Treatise on Madness*. London: Whiston and White.

Baudrillard, J. (1970) *La Société de Consommation: Ses Mythes, Ses Structures* [The Consumer Society: Myths and Structures]. Paris: Denoël.

Bauerlein, M. (2008) *The Dumbest Generation: How the Digital Age Stupefies Young Americans and Jeopardizes Our Future (Or, Don't Trust Anyone Under 30)*. New York: Tarcher/Penguin.

Bauman, Z. (2007) *Liquid Times: Living in an Age of Uncertainty*. Cambridge: Polity Press.

Bayle, A. L. J. (1826) *Traité des Maladies du Cerveau et de ses Membranes* [*Treatise on Diseases of the Brain and its Membranes*]. Paris: Chez Gabon et Compagnie Libraires.

BBC News (2012a) Prosecutors in Norway Call for Breivik Insanity Verdict. 21st June. www.bbc.co.uk/news/world-europe-18530670

BBC News (2012b) Anders Behring Breivik: Norway Court Finds Him Sane. 24th August. www.bbc.co.uk/news/world-europe-19365616. [accessed 26th October, 2015].

BBC News (2013) Stephen Fry Reveals He Attempted Suicide in 2012. www.bbc.co.uk/news/entertainment-arts-22782913. [accessed 2nd May, 2015].

Bean, P. (2008) *Madness and Crime*. Cullompton: Willan.

Bean, P., and Mounser, P. (1995) *Discharged from Mental Hospitals*. London: Mind.

Benes, F., and Berretta, S. (2001) GABAergic Interneurons: Implications for Understanding Schizophrenia and Bipolar Disorder. *Neuropsychopharmacology*, 25, pp. 1–27.

Bentall, R. (2003) *Madness Explained: Psychosis and Human Nature*. London: Allen Lane.

Bentall, R. (2009a) *Doctoring the Mind: Why Psychiatric Treatments Fail*. London: Penguin.

Bentall, R. (2009b) Formulating Zeppi: In: Sturmey, P. (Editor) *A Commentary. Clinical Case Formulation: Varieties of Approaches*. Chichester; Wiley. Chapter 9, pp. 119–131.

Bentall, R. (2011) One on One … with Richard Bentall. *The Psychologist*, 24, p.320.

Berger, P. L., and Luckmann, T. (1966) *The Social Construction of Reality: A Treatise in the Sociology of Knowledge*. New York: Anchor Books.

Berke, J. (2001) Epilogue. http://www.mary-barnes.co.uk/epiloque.htm. [accessed 19th January, 2016].

Berke, J. (2012) *Why I Hate You and You Hate Me. The Interplay of Envy, Greed, Jealousy and Narcissism in Everyday Life*. London: Karnac Books.

Berke, J. (2013) Joe Discussing Work of Mary Barnes at ART in ASYLUM Exhibition in Nottingham [video]. https://youtu.be/ljpDsk8o7O0 [accessed 14th April, 2014].

Berlin, I. (2003) The Salpêtrière Hospital: From Confining the Poor to Freeing the Insane. *American Journal of Psychiatry*, 160 (A68), p.1579.

Berrios, G. (1996) *The History of Mental Symptoms: Descriptive Psychopathology since the Nineteenth Century*. Cambridge: Cambridge University.

Besley, A. (2002) Foucault and the Turn to Narrative Therapy. *British Journal of Guidance and Counselling*, 30(2), pp. 125–143.

Bhaskar, R. (1975) *A Realist Theory of Science*. London: Verso.

Bhaskar, R. (2008) (interviewed by Hartwig, M.) *The Formation of Critical Realism: A Personal Perspective*. London: Routledge.

Bipolar UK (2016) Bi-polar – Frequently Asked Questions: The Facts. www.bipolaruk.org.uk/. [accessed 25th January, 2016].

Black, E. (2012) *War Against the Weak: Eugenics and America's Campaign to Create a Master Race*. Westport, CT: Dialog Press.

Blackburn, S. (2006) *Truth: A Guide for the Perplexed*. London: Penguin.

Blair, J., Mitchell, D., and Blair, K. (2005). *The Psychopath: Emotion and the Brain*. Oxford: Blackwell.

Bleuler, E. (1950; original 1911) *Dementia Praecox or the Group of Schizophrenias*. Translated by Zinkin, J. New York: International Universities Press.

Bocock, R. (2002) (second edition) *Sigmund Freud*. London: Routledge.

Boddy, J. (1994) Spirit Possession Revisited: Beyond Instrumentality. *Annual Review of Anthropology*, 23, pp. 407–434.

Bonn, S. (2014) How to Tell a Sociopath from a Psychopath: Understanding Important Distinctions, Between Criminal Sociopaths and Psychopaths. *Psychology Today*, 22nd January. www.psychologytoday.com/blog/wicked-deeds/201401/how-tell-sociopath-psychopath. [accessed 26th October, 2015].

Bonnie, R. (2002) Political Abuse of Psychiatry in the Soviet Union and in China: Complexities and Controversies. *Journal of American Academic Psychiatry Law*, 30, pp. 136–144.

Borchgrevink, A. (2012) *En Norsk Tragedie: Anders Behring Breivik og veiene til Utøya* [*A Norwegian Tragedy. Anders Behring Breivik and the Massacre on Utøya*]. Oslo: Gyldendal Norsk Forlag.

Boyle, M. (2002) (second edition) *Schizophrenia: A Scientific Delusion*. London: Routledge.

Breggin, R. (2007) (second edition) *Brain-Disabling Treatments in Psychiatry. Drugs, Electroshock, and the Psychopharmaceutical Complex*. New York: Springer.

Briggs, D. (2012) (editor) *The English Riots of 2011: A Summer of Discontent*. Hook: Waterside.

Broadgreen Pictures (2016). *Brain of Fire*. www.brainonfiremovie.com/. [accessed 24th March, 2016].

Brodie, R. (2009) *Virus of the Mind: The Revolutionary New Science of the Meme and How It Can Help You*. London: Hay House UK.

Brown, J. (2008) R D Laing: The Celebrity Shrink who put the Psychedelia into Psychiatry. *The Independent*, 29th September.

Brown, P. (1985) *Transfer of Care*. London: Routledge and Kegan Paul.

Brune, M. (2008) *Textbook of Evolutionary Psychiatry*. Oxford; Oxford University Press.

Buchanan, I. (2008) *The Anti-Oedipus: Capitalism and Schizophrenia*. London: Continuum.

Bunting, M. (2005) *Willing Slaves: How the Overwork Culture Is Ruling Our Lives*. New York: Harper Perennial.

Burnett, T. (2015) What is Scientism? *American Association for the Advancement of Science*. www.aaas.org/page/what-scientism. [accessed 2nd March 2016].

Burston, D. (1996) *The Wing of Madness: The Life and Work of R D Laing*. Cambridge, MA: Harvard University Press.

Burton, N. (2009) *The Meaning of Madness*. Oxford: Acheron.

Burton, R. (2004, original 1624) *The Anatomy of Melancholy: A Selection* (edited by Jackson, K.). Manchester: Carcanet.

Busfield, J. (1986) *Managing Madness: Changing Ideas and Practice*. London: Unwin Hyman.

Busfield, J. (1996) *Men, Women and Madness*. Basingstoke: Macmillan.

Busfield, J. (2011) *Mental Illness*. Cambridge: Polity.

Buss, D. (2005) *The Murderer Next Door: Why the Mind is Designed to Kill*. New York: Penguin.

Buss, D. (2014) *Evolutionary Psychology: The New Science of the Mind* (fifth edition). London: Routledge.

Buti, L. (2001) Italian Psychiatric Reform 20 Plus Years After. *Acta Psychiatrica Scandinavica*, 104 (Suppl. 410), pp. 41–46.

Butler, C., and Zeman, A. (2015) Neurological Syndromes Which can be Mistaken for Psychiatric Conditions. *Journal of Neurology, Neurosurgery and Psychiatry*, 76 (supplement 1), pp. 31–38.

Bynum, W., Porter, R., and Shepherd, M. (1988) (editors) *The Anatomy of Madness: Essays in the History of Psychiatry*, Volume 3. London: Routledge.

Cacioppo, J., and Berntson, G. (1992) Social Psychological Contributions to the Decade of the Brain: Doctrine of Multilevel Analysis. *American Psychologist*, 47(8), pp. 1019–1028.

Cadwallader, S. (2013) Susannah Cahalan: 'What I remember Most Vividly Are the Fear and Anger'. *The Guardian*, 13th January.

Cahalan, S. (2012a) *Brain on Fire: My Month of Madness*. London: Penguin.

Cahalan S (2012b) Susannah Cahalan's Month of Madness. YouTube. www.youtube.com/watch?v=Najj0aVLJwU. [accessed 30th November, 2016].

Cahalan, S. (2013) Susannah Cahalan at TEDxAmsterdamWomen 2013. YouTube. www.youtube.com/watch?v=oqrzvYnrI9A. [accessed 24th February, 2016].

Campling, P and Haigh, R. (1999) *Therapeutic Communities: Past, Present and Future.* London: Jessica Kingsley.

Carlson, N. (2009) Reviving Witiko (Windigo): An Ethnohistory of 'Cannibal Monsters' in the Athabasca District of Northern Alberta, 1878–1910. *Ethnohistory*, 56(3), pp. 55–394.

Carr, N. (2011) *The Shallows: What the Internet Is Doing to Our Brains.* London: Norton & Company.

CBS (2012) Stephen Fry: Renaissance Man – Without Tights. [television interview with Charlie Rose] www.cbsnews.com/news/stephen-fry-renaissance-man-without-tights/. [accessed 21st March, 2014].

Chadwick, P. (1997) *Schizophrenia: The Positive Persepctive.* London: Routledge.

Chan, D., and Sireling, L. (2010) I Want to be Bipolar – a New Phenomenon. *The Psychiatrist*, 34, pp. 103–105.

Chandler, D. (1976) *Capital Punishment in Canada.* Toronto: McClelland and Stewart.

Chapman, G., Palin, M., Cleese, J., Jones, T., Gilliam, T., and Idle, E. (2001) *The Monty Python's Life of Brian (of Nazareth).* (Screenplay.) York; Methuen.

Charle, C. (1994) (English edition; translated by Kochan, M.) *A Social History of France in the 19th Century.* Oxford: Berg.

Chiaburu, D., Thundiyil, T., and Wang, J. (2014) Alienation and its Correlates: A Meta-analysis. *European Management Journal*, 32(1), pp. 24-36.

Clark, D. (1975) *Social Therapy in Psychiatry.* New York: Jason Aronson.

Clinard, M., and Meire, R. (2016) (15th edition) *Sociology of Deviant Behavior.* Boston: Cengage.

Cockerham, W. (2007) *Social Causes of Health and Disease.* Cambridge: Polity.

Cockerham, W. (2013) (ninth edition) *Sociology of Mental Disorder.* New York: Routledge.

Cohen, B. (2016) *Psychiatric Hegemony: A Marxist Theory of Mental Illness.* London: Palgrave Macmillan.

Cohen, H. (1997) *Existential Thought and Therapeutic Practice: An Introduction to Existential Psychotherapy.* London: Sage.

Cohen, S., and Taylor, L. (1992) (second edition) *Escape Attempts: The Theory and Practice of Resistance in Everyday Life.* London: Routledge.

Cole, G. (1973) *Introduction Jean-Jacques Rousseau – The Social Contract and Discourses.* London: Dent.

Connor, S. (2015) Many People Have Genes Missing but are still Fit and Healthy. *The Guardian*, 1st October.

Conrad, P., and Schneider, J. (1980) *Deviance and Medicalisation: From Badness to Sickness.* St. Louis, MI: Mosby.

Cook, J., Nuccitelli, D., Green, S., Richardson, M., Winkler, B., Painting, R., Way, R. P., Jacobs, P., and Skuce, A. (2013) Quantifying the Consensus on Anthropogenic Global Warming in the Scientific Literature. *Environmental Research Letters*, 8(2). http://iopscience.iop.org/1748-9326/8/2/024024/article. [accessed 2nd May, 2015].

Cooper, D. (1967) *Psychiatry and Anti-psychiatry.* London: Tavistock.

Cooper, D. (1968) (editor) *The Dialectics of Liberation.* Harmondsworth: Penguin.

Cooper, J. M. (1933) The Cree Witiko Psychosis. *Primitive Man, Quarterly Bulletin of the Catholic Anthropological Conference*, 6(1), pp. 20–24.

Cooper, R. (2010) Are Culture-bound Syndromes as Real as Universally-occurring Disorders? *Studies in History and Philosophy of Science Part C: Studies in History and Philosophy of Biological and Biomedical Sciences*, 41(4), pp. 325–332.

Cooper, R., Kennelly, J., and Orduñez-Garcia, P. (2006) Health in Cuba. *International Journal of Epidemiology*, 35 (4), pp. 817–824.

Coppock, V. and Hopton, J. (2000) *Critical Perspectives on Mental Health*. London: Routledge.

Costello, P. (2014) My Rendezvous with Insanity – A Conversation with Susannah Cahalan. *Stanford Medicine Magazine*, 23rd October. https://neuroscience.stanford.edu/news/my-rendezvous-insanity-conversation-susannah-cahalan. [accessed 24th February, 2016].

Cox, J. (1986) *Transcultural Psychiatry*. London: Routledge.

Credit Suisse (2015) *Global Wealth Report 2015*. Zurich: Credit Suisse.

Cross-Disorder Group of the Psychiatric Genomics Consortium (2013) Identification of Risk Loci with Shared Effects on Five Major Psychiatric Disorders: A Genome-wide Analysis. *Lancet*, April 20th, 381(9875), pp. 1371–1379.

Darwin, C. (1859) *On The Origin Of Species By Means Of Natural Selection, Or The Preservation Of Favoured Races In The Struggle For Life*. London: Murray.

Darwin, C., and Russel, W. A. (1858) On the Tendency of Species to form Varieties; and on the Perpetuation of Varieties and Species by Natural Means of Selection. *Zoological Journal of the Linnean Society*, 3, pp. 46–50.

Davies, H. (2010) *The Financial Crisis: Who is to Blame?* Cambridge: Polity.

Davies, J. (2013) *Cracked: Why Psychiatry is Doing More Harm Than Good*. London: Icon.

Davis, M. (2013) *Voices from the Asylum: West Riding Pauper Lunatic Asylum*. Stroud: Amberley.

Dawkins, R. (1976) *The Selfish Gene*. Oxford: Oxford University Press.

Dawkins, R. (2006) *The God Delusion*. London: Bantam Press.

Dawkins, R. (2013) *An Appetite for Wonder: The Making of a Scientist*. London: Bantam.

Dawkins, R. (2015) *Brief Candle in the Dark: My Life in Science*. London: Bantam.

Day, E. (2008) He [Howard Dully] was Bad, so they Put an Ice Pick in his Brain … *The Observer*, 13th January.

Day, E., Keeley, G., and Toms, K. (2008) 'Dad [R D Laing] Solved Other People's Problems – But Not His Own'. *The Observer*, 1st June.

Deacon, B. (2013) The Biomedical Model of Mental Disorder: A Critical Analysis of its Validity, Utility, and Effects on Psychotherapy Research. *Clinical Psychology Review*, 33(7), pp. 846–861.

Deery, S., Iverson, R., and Walsh, J. (2002) Work Relationships in Telephone Call Centres: Understanding Emotional Exhaustion and Employee Withdrawal. *Journal of Management Studies*, 39(4), pp. 471–496.

Dellar, R., Curtis, T. and Leslie, E. (editors) (2000) *Mad Pride*. London: Chipmunka.

Dennis, D., Buckner, J., and Lipton, F. (1991) A Decade of Research and Services for Homeless Mentally Ill Persons: Where do we Stand? *American Psychologist*, 46(11), pp. 1129–1138.

Department of Health (2015) New Social Contract between the Public, Health and Care Services. 1st July. www.gov.uk/government/news/new-social-contract-between-the-public-health-and-care-services. [accessed 25th November, 2015].

Derrida, J. (1967) *De la grammatologie* [*Of Grammatology*]. Paris: Editions de Minuit.

Descartes, R. (1637) *Discours de la Méthode. Discours de la méthode pour bien conduire sa raison et chercher la vérité dans les sciences* [*Discourse on the Method of Rightly Conducting the Reason and Seeking Truth in the Sciences*]. Paris (1668 edition): Bobin & le Gras.

Descartes, R. (1644) *Principia Philosophiae* [*Principles of Philosophy*]. Amsterdam (1677 edition): Elsevier.

DigitalSpy (2012) Stephen Fry is the Celebrity that most Brits Would Want as PM. www.digitalspy.co.uk/showbiz/news/a359716/stephen-fry-is-the-celebrity-that-most-brits-would-want-as-pm.html. [accessed 11th December, 2014].

Dimofte, C., Haugtvedt, C., and Yalch, R. (2015) *Consumer Psychology in a Social Media World*. London: Routledge.

Domhoff, G. W. (2014) (seventh edition) *Who Rules America? The Triumph of the Corporate Rich*. Maidenhead; McGraw-Hill.

Double, D. (editor) (2006) *Critical Psychiatry. The Limits of Madness*. Basingstoke: Palgrave Macmillan.

Doward, J. (2013) Psychiatrists Under Fire in Mental Health Battle: British Psychological Society to Launch Attack on Rival Profession, Casting Doubt on Biomedical Model of Mental Illness. *The Observer*, 12th May.

Dowbiggin, I. (1997) *Keeping America Sane: Psychiatry and Eugenics in the United States and Canada, 1880–1940*. New York: Cornell University Press.

Dreyfus, H. (1987) Foucault's Critique of Psychiatric Medicine. *Journal of Medical Philosophy*, 12(4), pp. 311–333.

Dully, H., and Fleming, C. (2008) *Messing With My Head: The Shocking True Story of My Lobotomy*. New York: Vermillion.

Durkheim, E. (2013; original 1895) *The Rules of Sociological Method and Selected Texts on Sociology and its Method* [edited by Lukes, S.]. London: Palgrave.

Dyck, E. (2008) *Psychedelic Psychiatry: LSD from Clinic to Campus*. Baltimore, MD: Johns Hopkins University Press.

Eagleman, D. (2015) *The Brain: The Story of You*. Edinburgh: Canongate.

[The] *Economist* (2015) The Social Contract: Special issue, Singapore. 18th July. www.economist.com/news/special-report/21657613-two-big-simple-government-promisesof-home-and-comfortable-old-agehave-become-harder. [accessed 25th November, 2015].

Eisenberg, L. (1977) Psychiatry and Society: A Sociobiologic Synthesis. *New England Journal of Medicine*, 296(16), pp. 903–910.

Eisenberg, L. (1986) Mindlessness and Brainlessness in Psychiatry. *The British Journal of Psychiatry*, 148(5), pp. 497–508.

Eisenberg, L., and Kleinman, A. (1980) (editors) *The Relevance of Social Science for Medicine*. New York: Springer.

Emmott, S. (2013) *Ten Billion*. London: Penguin.

Engels, F. (1969, original 1845) *The Condition of the Working Class in England*. St. Albans: Granada.

Ernst, E. (2015) *A Scientist in Wonderland: A Memoir of Searching for Truth and Finding Trouble*. Exeter: Imprint Academic

Esterson, A. (2015) Psychoanalysis, Their Weird Theories – Neuroscience & Freud. Freud Returns? www.skeptically.org/minther/id5.html. [accessed 20th February, 2015].

Esquirol E (1838) *Des Maladies Mentales: Considérées Sous les Rapports Médical, Hygiénique et Médico-légal*. Paris: Baillière.

Esquirol, E. (1845) (translated from original French edition by Hunt, E.) *Mental Maladies: Treatise on Insanity*. Philadelphia, PA: Lea and Blanchard.

Etsuko, M. (1991) The Interpretations of Fox Possession: Illness as Metaphor. *Culture, Medicine and Psychiatry*, 15, pp. 453–477.

Fallon, J. (2014) How I Discovered I Have the Brain of a Psychopath. *The Guardian*, 3rd June. www.theguardian.com/commentisfree/2014/jun/03/how-i-discovered-i-have-the-brain-of-a-psychopath. [accessed 30th September, 2015].

Faris, R., and Dunham, W. (1965). *Mental Disorders in Urban Areas*. Chicago, IL: University of Chicago Press.

Featherstone, S. (2005) *Post-Colonial Cultures*. Edinburgh: Edinburgh University Press.

Feist, J., Feist, G., and Roberts, T. (2017) (9th edition) *Theories of Personality*. Columbus, OH: McGraw-Hill.

Feldman, G. (2008) *Cannibalism, Headhunting and Human Sacrifice in North America: A History Forgotten*. Chambersburg, PA: Alan C Hood & Company.

Feltham, C. (2007) *What's Wrong with Us?: The Anthropathology Thesis*. Chichester: Wiley.

Feltham, C. (2014) Whatever Happened to Critical Thinking? *Therapy Today*, 25(3), www.therapytoday.net/article/show/4221/whatever-happened-to-critical-thinking/. [accessed 20th April, 2015].

Felthous, A., and Sass, H. (2007) (editors) *The International Handbook on Psychopathic Disorders Volume 1*. Chichester; Wiley.

Fennell, P. (1996) *Treatment Without Consent: Law, Psychiatry and the Treatment of Mentally Disordered People Since 1845*. London: Routledge.

Feresin, E. (2009) Lighter Sentence for Murderer with 'Bad Genes': Italian Court Reduces Jail Term After Tests Identify Genes Linked to Violent Behaviour. *Nature*, 30th October. www.nature.com/news/2009/091030/full/news.2009.1050.html?s=news_rss. [accessed 9th February, 2016].

Feuer, L. (1978) (editor) *Marx and Engels: Basic Writings on Politics and Philosophy*. Glasgow: Fontana/Collins.

Fibiger, C. (2012) Psychiatry, The Pharmaceutical Industry, and The Road to Better Therapeutics. *Schizophrenia Bulletin*, 38(4), pp. 649–650.

Fisher, C. (2014) Psychiatry's New Surgeons. *Scientific American Mind*, 25(1), pp. 24–25.

Fletcher, N. (2008) Hyperactivity Drug Goes Too Slow for Shire. *The Guardian*, Wednesday 7th May.

Forcen, F. (2013) Father Jofre and the Founding of the First Insane Asylum. *Journal of Humanistic Psychiatry*, 1(1), pp. 9–11.

Foth, G. (2013) *Caring and Killing – the Participation of German Nurses in the Nazi Euthanasia Programme*. Göttingen: V&R Unipress, Universitätsverlag Osnabrück.

Foucault, M. (1961) *Folie et Déraison: Histoire de la folie à l'âge classique* [retitled in English as *Madness and Civilization*, New York, 1965]. Paris: Librarie Plon.

Foucault, M. (1963) *Naissance de la Clinique*. [*Birth of the Clinic*] Paris: Universitaires de France.

Foucault, M. (1966) *Les mots et les choses: Une archéologie des science* [*The Order of Things: An Archaeology of the Human Sciences*]. Paris: Gaillimard

Foucault, M. (1975) (editor) *I, Pierre Riviere, Having Slaughtered My Mother, My Sister and My Brother: A Case of Parricide in the 19th Century* [Translated by Jellinek, F. from original, *Moi, Pierre Riviere ayant egorgé ma mere, ma soeur et mon frere*, 1973, Editions Gallimard/Julliard]. New York: Pantheon.

Foucault, M. (1988) The Dangerous Individual. In Kritzman, L. (editor) *Michel Foucault: Politics, Philosophy, Culture: Interviews and Other Writings of Michel Foucault, 1977–1984*. New York: Routledge, Chapter 8, pp. 125–151.

Foucault, M. (2006) *Psychiatric Power: Lectures at the Collège de France*. Basingstoke: Palgrave Macmillan.

Frances, A. (2010) Opening Pandora's Box: The 19 Worst Suggestions For DSM5. *Psychiatric Times*, 11th February, 27(2). www.psychiatrictimes.com/dsm/content/article/10168/1522341. [accessed 11th January, 2014].

Frances, A. (2013a) The Past, Present and Future of Psychiatric Diagnosis. *World Psychiatry*, 12(2), pp. 111–112.

Frances, A. (2013b) Bad News: DSM 5 Refuses to Correct Somatic Symptom Disorder – Medical Illness Will be Mislabeled Mental Disorder. *Psychology Today*, 16th January, www.psychologytoday.com/blog/dsm5-in-distress/201301/bad-news-dsm-5-refuses-correct-somatic-symptom-disorder. [accessed 10th January, 2014].

Frances, A. (2014) *Saving Normal: An Insider's Revolt Against Out-Of-Control Psychiatric Diagnosis, DSM-5, Big Pharma, and the Medicalization of Ordinary Life*. New York: William Morrow.

Franzen, C. (2008) Syphilis in Composers and Musicians – Mozart, Beethoven, Paganini, Schubert, Schumann, Smetana. *European Journal of Clinical Microbiology and Infectious Diseases*, 27(12), pp. 1151–1157.

Freud, S. (1905) *Drei Abhandlungen zur Sexualtheorie [Three Essays on the Theory of Sexuality]*. Leipzig: Deuticke.

Freud, S. (1914) Zur Einführung des Narzißmus [On Narcissism: An Introduction]. In Strachey, J. (2001) (editor) *The Standard Edition of the Complete Psychological Works of Sigmund Freud*. London: Vintage.

Freud, S. (1920) Jenseits des Lustprinzips [Beyond the Pleasure Principle]. In Strachey, J. (2001) (editor) *The Standard Edition of the Complete Psychological Works of Sigmund Freud*. London: Vintage.

Freud, S. (1923) German: Das Ich und das Es [The Ego and the Id]. In Strachey, J. (2001) (editor) *The Standard Edition of the Complete Psychological Works of Sigmund Freud*. London: Vintage.

Freud, S. (1930) Das Unbehagen in der Kultur [The Uneasiness in Culture; later published in English: Civilization and Its Discontents]. In Strachey, J. (2001) (editor) *The Standard Edition of the Complete Psychological Works of Sigmund Freud*. London: Vintage.

Friedi, L. (2009) *Mental Health, Resilience and Inequalities*. Copenhagen: World Health Organization.

Friedman, L. (2013) *The Lives of Erich Fromm: Love's Prophet*. New York: Columbia University Press.

Frith, J. (2012) Syphilis – Its Early History and Treatment until Penicillin and the Debate on its Origins. *Journal of Military and Veterans' Health (Australia)*, 20(4). http://jmvh.org/article/syphilis-its-early-history-and-treatment-until-penicillin-and-the-debate-on-its-origins/. [accessed 30th October, 2015].

Fromm, E. (1939) Selfishness and Self-Love. *Journal for the Study of Interpersonal Process* Vol. 2, pp. 507–523.

Fromm, E. (1955) *The Sane Society*. New York: Rinehart.

Fry, S. (2004) *Moab Is My Washpot*. London: Arrow.

Fry, S. (2010) Stephen Fry on Manic Depression [YouTube recording] www.youtube.com/watch?v=cKiAz6ndUbU [accessed 29th January, 2014].

Fry, S. (2011) *The Fry Chronicles*. London: Penguin.

Fry, S. (2013) An Open Letter to David Cameron and Members of the IOC [International Olympic Committee]. www.stephenfry.com/2013/08/07/an-open-letter-to-david-cameron-and-the-ioc/ [accessed 26th March, 2014].

Fry, S. (2014) How Can I be Happy? YouTube. [video]. www.youtube.com/watch?v=Tvz0mmF6NW4. [accessed 10th December, 2014].

Fry, S. (2015) *More Fool Me: A Memoir*. London: Penguin.

Fuller, S. (2014) *Science (The Art of Living)*. London: Routledge.

Fund for Peace. Fragile States Index 2015. http://fsi.fundforpeace.org/. [accessed 26th November, 2015].

Fuster, J. (2013) *The Neuroscience of Freedom and Creativity: Our Predictive Brain*. Cambridge: Cambridge University Press.

Gabbard, G. (2009) (editor) *Textbook of Psychotherapeutic Treatments*. Arlington, VA: American Psychiatric Association.

Gajilan, A. C. (2005) Survivor Recounts Lobotomy at Age 12. CNN [Television, USA]. December 1st. http://edition.cnn.com/2005/HEALTH/conditions/11/30/pdg.lobotomy/ [accessed 5th November, 2015].

Gallagher, J., Buchanan, R., and Luck-Baker, A. (2016) Depression: A Revolution in Treatment? [*The Inflamed Mind*, BBC Radio 4 programme] www.bbc.co.uk/news/health-37166293 [accessed 25th August, 2016].

Gates Foundation (2015) Foundation Fact Sheet. www.gatesfoundation.org/Who-We-Are/General-Information/Foundation-Factsheet. [accessed 29th January, 2016].

Géraud, M. (2007) Emil Kraepelin: A Pioneer of Modern Psychiatry: On the Occasion of the Hundred and Fiftieth Anniversary of his Birth. *Encephale* 33(4), pp. 561–567.

Gibney, P. (2006) The Double Bind Theory: Still Crazy-Making After All These Years. *Psychotherapy in Australia*, 12(3), 48–55.

Giddens, A. (1991) *Modernity and Self-identity: Self and Society in the Late Modern Age.* Cambridge: Polity Press.

Giddens, A. (2009) *Sociology*. Cambridge: Polity.

Giddens, A., and Sutton, P. (2013) *Sociology*. Cambridge: Polity.

Gilburt, H. (2015) *Mental Health Under Pressure*: King's Fund Briefing, London: Kings Fund.

Gillen, M. (1972) *Assassination of the Prime Minister: Shocking Death of Spencer Perceval.* London: Sidgwick & Jackson.

Gittins, D. (1998) *Madness in its Place: Narratives of Severalls Hospital.* London: Routledge.

Goetz, C. (1999) Charcot and the Myth of Misogyny. *Neurology*, 52(8), pp. 1678–1686.

Goffman, E. (1959) *The Presentation of Self in Everyday Life.* New York: Anchor.

Goffman, E. (1961) *Asylums: Essays on the Social Situation of Mental Patients and Other Inmates.* New York: Anchor.

Goffman, E. (1963) *Stigma: Notes on the Management of Spoiled Identity.* Harmondsworth: Penguin.

Goldacre, B. (2007) Pink, Pink, Pink. Pink Moan. *The Guardian*, 25th August.

Goldacre, B. (2009) *Bad Science.* London: Harper Perennial.

Goldacre, B. (2012) *Bad Pharma: How Drug Companies Mislead Doctors and Harm Patients.* London: Fourth Estate.

Goodenough, O., and Zeki, S. (2006) *Law and the Brain.* Oxford: Oxford University Press.

Goodwin, B. (2007) *Nature's Due: Healing Our Fragmented Culture.* Edinburgh: Floris.

Google (2016) Stephen Fry. www.google.co.uk. [accessed 1st October, 2016].

Gordon, B. (2010) Stephen Fry is in No Position to Comment on Women's Sex Lives. *The Telegraph,* 1st November.

Gore, A. (2006) *An Inconvenient Truth: The Planetary Emergency of Global Warming and What We Can Do About It.* Emmaus, Philadelphia, PA: Rodale.

Gould, S. J. (1997) Darwinian Fundamentalism. *New York Review of Books*, 12th June. www.nybooks.com/articles/archives/1997/jun/12/darwinian-fundamentalism/?page=1. [accessed 2nd July, 2014].

Gray, S. (1995) *Fat Chance: 'Stephen Fry Quits' Drama.* London: Faber & Faber.

Greenberg, G. (2014) *The Book of Woe: The DSM and the Unmaking of Psychiatry.* New York: Plume.

Greenfield, S. (2016) *Day in the Life of the Brain: The Neuroscience of Consciousness from Dawn Till Dusk.* London: Allen Lane.

Greenhalgh, T., and Wessely, S. (2004) 'Health For Me': A Sociocultural Analysis of Healthism in the Middle Classes. *British Medical Bulletin*, 69, pp. 197–213.

Greer, G. (1970) *The Female Eunuch.* New York: Bantam.

Gribbin, J. (2003) *Science: A History 1534–2001.* London: Penguin.

Griesinger, W. (1882; original 1867) (second edition) *Mental Pathology and Therapeutics* [translated by Robertson, L., and Rutherford, J.]. New York: Wood & Co.

Griffiths, A. (2014) Stephen Fry STILL in Front as Twitter Survey Reveals Brits Obsessed with Tweeting Celebrities. *Daily Mirror,* 29th July.

Grimes, W. (2007) Spikes in the Brain, and a Search for Answers. *New York Times*, 14th September. www.nytimes.com/2007/09/14/books/14book.html?_r=0. [accessed 11th November, 2013].

[The] Guardian (2014) Norwegian Mass Murderer Anders Breivik's Father to Publish Book: Jens Breivik's My Fault? 20th August.

Gullestad, S. E. (2013) Ideological Destructiveness: A Psychoanalytic Perspective on the Massacre of July 22, 2011. *American Psychological Association – Psychoanalysis Division*. www.apadivisions.org/division-39/publications/review/2013/04/ideological-destructiveness.asp. [accessed 5th August, 2014].

Haas, L. (1997) Neurological Stamp: Wilhelm Griesinger (1817–68). *Journal of Neurology, Neurosurgery, and Psychiatry*, 62(5): 435.

Hacker, P. (2015) Philosophy and Scientism: What Cognitive Neuroscience Can and Cannot Explain. In: Robinson, D., and Williams, R. (editors) *Scientism: The New Orthodoxy*. London: Bloomsbury. Chapter, 5, pp. 97–116.

Hagerty, B. (2010, 29th June) A Neuroscientist Uncovers A Dark Secret. NPR [public radio, USA]. www.npr.org/templates/story/story.php?storyId=127888976. [accessed 14th March, 2014].

Hales, R., Yudofsky, S., and Roberts, L. (2014) *The American Psychiatric Publishing Textbook of Psychiatry*. Arlington, VA: American Psychiatric Publishing.

Hanhimäki, J., and Blumenau, B. (2013) (editors) *An International History of Terrorism: Western and Non-Western Experiences*. London: Routledge.

Hanrahan, D. (2012) *The Assassination of the Prime Minister: John Bellingham and the Murder of Spencer Perceval*. Dursley: The History Press.

Hare, R. (1996) Psychopathy and Antisocial Personality Disorder: A Case of Diagnostic Confusion. *Psychiatric Times*, 1st February, 13(2). www.psychiatrictimes.com/antisocial-personality-disorder/psychopathy-and-antisocial-personality-disorder-case-diagnostic-confusion/page/0/1#sthash.N0FD6kbg.dpuf [accessed 20th October, 2015].

Hare, R. (1999) *Without Conscience: The Disturbing World of the Psychopaths Among Us*. New York: Guilford Press.

Hare, R. (2003) (second edition) *Manual for the Revised Psychopathy Checklist*. Toronto, Ontario: Multi-Health Systems.

Haslam, J. (1798) *Observations on Insanity, with Practical Remarks on the Disease, and an Account of the Morbid Appearances on Dissection*. London: Rivington.

Hatch, E. (1983) *Culture and Morality: The Relativity of Values in Anthropology*. New York: Columbia University Press.

Haussmann, R., Bauer, M., von Bonin, S., Grof, P., and Lewitzka, U. (2015) Treatment of Lithium Intoxication: Facing the Need for Evidence. *International Journal of Bipolar Disorders*, 3(23). http://journalbipolardisorders.springeropen.com/articles/10.1186/s40345-015-0040-2. [accessed 25th January, 2016].

Hazelton, M., and Morrall, P. (2016) Mental Health, the Law and Human Rights. In: Chambers, M. (editor; third edition) *Psychiatric and Mental Health Nursing: The Craft of Caring*. London: Hodder & Arnold.

Helman, C. (2006) *Suburban Shaman: Tales from Medicine's Front Line*. London: Hammersmith Press.

Helman, C. (2007) (fifth edition) *Culture, Health and Illness*. London: Hodder Arnold.

Herald-Scotland (2009) RD Laing Beat Me Up, Claims Daughter, 13th April. www.heraldscotland.com/rd-laing-beat-me-up-claims-daughter-1.907408 [accessed 23rd April, 2015].

Hirst, P., and Woolley, P. (1982) *Social Relations and Human Attributes*. London: Tavistock.

Hitchens, C. (2007) *God Is Not Great: The Case Against Religion*. London: Atlantic Books.

Hodgkin, K. (2006) *Madness in Seventeenth-century Autobiography*. Basingstoke: Palgrave Macmillan.

Holmwood, J. (2005) Functionalism and its Critics. In: Harrington, A. (editor) *Modern Social Theory: An Introduction*. Oxford: Oxford University Press, Chapter 4, pp. 87–109.

Honberg, R., Diehl, S., Kimball, A., Gruttadaro, D., and Fitzpatrick, M. (2011) *State Mental Health Cuts: A National Crisis*. Arlington, VA: National Alliance on Mental Illness.

Hook, D. (2010) *Foucault, Psychology and the Analytics of Power: Critical Theory and Practice in Psychology and the Human Sciences*. London: Palgrave.

Horney, K. (1993) *Feminine Psychology*. New York: Norton.

Howard, T. (2014) (second edition) *Failed States and the Origins of Violence*. Farnham; Ashgate.

Howarth-Williams, M. (1977) *R.D. Laing: His Work and its Relevance for Sociology*. London: Routledge & Kegan Paul.

Hudson, C. (2005) Socioeconomic Status and Mental Illness: Tests of the Social Causation and Selection Hypotheses. *American Journal of Orthopsychiatry*, 75(1), pp. 3–18.

Huertas, R. (2008) Between Doctrine and Clinical Practice: Nosography and Semiology in the Work of Jean-Etienne-Dominique Esquirol (1772–1840). *History of Psychiatry*, 19 (2), pp. 123–140.

Hughes, J. (1991) (third edition) *An Outline of Modern Psychiatry*. Chichester: Wiley.

Hunt, T. (2010) *The Frock-Coated Communist: The Life and Times of the Original Champagne Socialist* [Friedrich Engels]. London: Penguin.

Hurn, J. D. (1998) *The History of General Paralysis of the Insane in Britain, 1830–1950*. PhD thesis. London: University College.

Husserl, E. (1970) (original 1936) *The Crises of European and Transcendental Phenomenology* [translated by Carr, D.]. Evanston, IL: Northwestern University Press.

Illich, I. (1975) *Medical Nemesis: The Expropriation of Health*. London: Marian Boyars.

Illich, I., Zola, I., and McKnight, J. (1977) *Disabling Professions*. London: Marion Boyars.

Insel, T. (2015) Psychiatry is Reinventing Itself Thanks to Advances in Biology. *New Scientist*, 3035, 19th August. www.newscientist.com/article/mg22730353-000-psychiatry-is-reinventing-itself-thanks-to-advances-in-biology/. [accessed 13th November, 2015].

Institute of Psychiatry, Psychology and Neuroscience (2015) *About the Institute: The Institute of Psychiatry, Psychology & Neuroscience*, King's College London. www.kcl.ac.uk/ioppn/about/index.aspx

Inta, D., Lang, U., Borgwardt, S., Meyer-Lindenberg, A., and Gass, P. (2016) Adult Neurogenesis in the Human Striatum: Possible Implications for Psychiatric Disorders. *Molecular Psychiatry [Nature]*, 21, pp. 446–447.

Intergovernmental Panel on Climate Change (2015) *Climate Change 2014 Report*. Geneva: Intergovernmental Panel on Climate Change.

International Criminal Court (2016) What are crimes against humanity? www.icc-cpi.int/en_menus/icc/about%20the%20court/frequently%20asked%20questions/Pages/12.asp. [accessed 5th January, 2016].

International Monetary Fund (2015) *Vulnerabilities, Legacies, and Policy Challenges. Risks Rotating to Emerging Markets*. Washington, DC: International Monetary Fund.

Ioannidis, J. (2005) Why Most Published Research Findings Are False. *PLOS Medicine*. 30th August. http://journals.plos.org/plosmedicine/article?id=10.1371/journal.pmed.0020124. [accessed 8th March, 2016].

Ioannidis, J. (2014) How to Make More Published Research True. *PLOS Medicne*, 21st October. http://journals.plos.org/plosmedicine/article?id=10.1371/journal.pmed.1001747. [accessed 8th March 2014].

Itten, T. (2012) R. D. Laing (1927–1989): A Biography. In: Itten, T. and Young, C. (editors) *R D Laing: Fifty Years Since the Divided Self*. Ross-on-Wye: PCCS. Chapter 28, pp. 315–319.

Itten, T., and Young, C. (2012) (editors) *R D Laing: Fifty Years Since the Divided Self*. Ross-on-Wye: PCCS.

Jacobsen, M., and Kristiansen, S. (2014) *The Social Thought of Erving Goffman*. London: Sage.

James, F. E. (1996) *The Life and Work of Thomas Laycock (1812–1876)*. PhD thesis. London: University of London.

James, O. (2007) *Afluenza*. London: Vermillion.

James, O. (2008) *The Selfish Capitalist*. London: Vermillion.

James, O. (2016) *Not In Your Genes: The Real Reasons Children are Like Their Parents*. London: Vermillion.

Jamison, K. R. (1993) *Touched with Fire: Manic Depressive Illness and the Artistic Temperament*. New York: Free Press.

Jamison, K. R. (1995) *An Unquiet Mind: A Memoir of Moods and Madness*. New York: Borzoi.

Johnstone, L. (2000) (second edition) *Users and Abusers of Psychiatry. A Critical Look at Psychiatric Practice*. London: Brunner-Routledge.

Johnstone, L. (2013) Quoted in Doward, J.: Psychiatrists Under Fire in Mental Health. *The Observer*, 12th May.

Johnstone, L. (2014) *A Straight Talking Introduction to Psychiatric Diagnosis*. Ross-on-Wye: PCCS.

Johnstone, L., and Dallos, R. (2006) *Formulation in Psychology and Psychotherapy: Making Sense of People's Problems*. London: Routledge.

Jones, J. H. (1993) *Bad Blood: Tuskegee Syphilis Experiment*. New York: Free Press.

Jones, M. (1953) *The Therapeutic Community: A New Treatment Method in Psychiatry*. New York: Basic Books.

Jung, C. (1970) *Psychoanalysis and Neurosis*. Princeton, NJ: Princeton University Press.

Kabria, A.,. and Metcalfe, N. (2014) A Biography of William Tuke (1732–1822): Founder of the Modern Mental Asylum. *Journal of Medical Biography*. June, 149(6). www.ncbi.nlm. nih.gov/pubmed/24944052.

Kahneman, D. (2011) *Thinking, Fast and Slow*. London: Penguin.

Kaplan, H., Sadock, B., and Grebb, J. (1996) (seventh edition) *Kaplan and Sadock's Synopsis of Psychiatry: Behavioral Sciences Clinical Psychiatry*. Baltimore, MD: Williams and Wilkins.

Kaplan, R. (2010) Syphilis, Sex and Psychiatry, 1789–1925: Part 1. *Australian Psychiatry*, 18(1), pp. 17–21.

Karban, K. (2011) *Social Work and Mental Health*. Cambridge: Polity.

Kay, J. (2015) *People's Money: Masters of the Universe or Servants of the People?* London: Profile.

Keller, R. (2007) *Colonial Madness: Psychiatry in French North Africa*. Chicago, IL: University of Chicago.

Kellner, C. (2011) Electroconvulsive Therapy: The Second Most Controversial Medical Procedure. *Psychiatric Times*, 28(1), 8th February. www.psychiatrictimes.com/major-depressive-disorder/electroconvulsive-therapy-second-most-controversial-medical-procedure. [accessed 5th November, 2015].

Kelly, J. (1984) (second edition) *Women, History, and Theory: The Essays of Joan Kelly*. Chicago, IL: University of Chicago.

Kerner, B. (2014) Genetics of Bipolar Disorder. *Applied Clinical Genetics*, 7(33), pp. 33–42.

Kety, S. (1974) From Rationalization to Reason. *American Journal of Psychiatry*, 131, pp. 957–963.

Kilvert, F. (1978) *Kilvert's Diary: Selections From the Diary of the Reverend Francis Kilvert 1870–1879* [edited by Plomer, W.]. London: Book Club Associates.

Kimonis, E. (2015) Insanity Defense/Guilty but Mentally Ill. *Encyclopedia of Clinical Psychology*, 23rd January. http://onlinelibrary.wiley.com/doi/10.1002/9781118625392. wbecp429/abstract?userIsAuthenticated=false&deniedAccessCustomisedMessage

King's College London (2016) Bethlem Royal Hospital. www.kcl.ac.uk/lsm/education/meded/clinicalcommunity/clusters/Denmark-Hill/brh.aspx. [accessed 15th August, 2016].

Klein, N. (2015) *This Changes Everything: Capitalism vs. the Climate*. London: Penguin.

Kleinman, A. (1987) Anthropology and Psychiatry. The Role of Culture in Cross-Cultural Research on Illness. *Psychiatry*, 151, pp. 447–454.

Kleinman, A. (1988) *Rethinking Psychiatry: From Cultural Category to Personal Experience*. New York: Free Press.

Knox, D., and Holloman, G. (2012) Use and Avoidance of Seclusion and Restraint: Consensus Statement of the American Association for Emergency Psychiatry Project BETA Seclusion and Restraint Workgroup. *Western Journal of Emergency Medicine*, 13(1), pp. 35–40.

Koić, E., Filaković, P., Nad, S., and Celić, I. (2005) Glossolalia. *Collegium Antropologicum*, 29(1), pp. 373–379.

Koven, S. (2015) *The Match Girl and the Heiress*. Princeton, NJ: Princeton University Press.

Kramer, P. (1994) *Listening to Prozac: A Psychiatrist Explores Antidepressant Drugs and Remaking of the Self*. London: Fourth Estate.

Kuhn, T. (1962) *The Structure of Scientific Revolutions*. Chicago, IL: University of Chicago. Press.

Laing, A. (1997) *R.D.Laing: A Biography*. New York: Harper Collins.

Laing, A. (2010) Amazon.co.uk review by Laing's son Adrian Laing of Szsasz's *Antipsychiatry: Quackery Squared*. 17th August. www.amazon.co.uk/Antipsychiatry-Quackery-Squared-Thomas-Szasz/dp/0815609434. [accessed 25th November, 2013].

Laing, R. D. (1960) *The Divided Self: An Existential Study in Sanity and Madness*. London: Tavistock.

Laing, R. D. (1967) *The Politics of Experience*. London: Routledge & Kegan Paul.

Laing, R. D. (1969) *Politics of the Family*. Toronto: Canadian Broadcasting Corporation.

Laing, R. D., and Cooper, D. (1964) *Reason and Violence: A Decade of Sartre's Philosophy 1950–1960*. London: Tavistock.

Laing, R. D., and Esterson, A. (1964) *Sanity, Madness and the Family*. London: Tavistock.

Lambert, M. (2002) (revised edition) *Medieval Heresy: Popular Movements from the Gregorian Reform to the Reformation*. Chichester; Wiley-Blackwell.

Landes, R. (1937) The Personality of the Ojibwa. *Character and Personality*, 6, pp. 51–60.

Landy, D. (1977) *Culture, Disease, and Healing: Studies in Medical Anthropology*. Edinburgh: Macmillan.

Lasch, C. (1979) *The Culture of Narcissism: American Life in an Age of Diminishing Expectations*. New York: Norton.

Lawson, M. (2016) The Healing Nature of Communion: Scottish Psychoanalysis, R.D. Laing, and Therapeutic Communities. *Journal of Theoretical and Philosophical Psychology*, 36(1), pp. 20–28.

Layard, R., and Clark, D. (2014) *Thrive: The Power of Evidence-Based Psychological Therapies*. London: Allen Lane.

Laycock, J. (2014) *Spirit Possession Around the World: Possession, Communion, and Demon Expulsion Across Cultures*. Santa Barbara, CA: ABC-CLIO.

Leach, E. (1967) Runaway World. BBC Reith Lecture, 1967. Transmitted 17 December 1967 on BBC Radio 4. http://downloads.bbc.co.uk/rmhttp/radio4/transcripts/1967_reith3.pdf. [accessed 26th November, 2013].

Leader, D. (2013) *Strictly Bipolar*. London: Penguin.

Leahy, R. (2011) Cognitive-Behavioral Therapy: Proven Effectiveness. *Psychology Today*. www.psychologytoday.com/blog/anxiety-files/201111/cognitive-behavioral-therapy-proven-effectiveness. [accessed 20th February, 2015].

Le Blanc, P. (2016) (second edition) *From Marx to Gramsci: A Reader in Revolutionary Marxist Politics*. Chicago, IL: Haymarket.

Leff, J. (2001) Why is Care in the Community Perceived as a Failure? *British Journal of Psychiatry*, 179(5), pp. 381–383.

Leseth, B. (2015) What is Culturally Informed Psychiatry? Cultural Understanding and Withdrawal in the Clinical Encounter. *British Journal of Psychiatry Bulletin*, 39(40), pp. 187–109.

Lewis, P. (2015) Assisted Dying: What Does the Law in Different Countries Say? www.bbc. co.uk/news/world-34445715. [accessed 22nd October, 2015].

Lexington, P. (2014) The Nostalgia Trap: Politicians Need to Stop Pretending to Angry Voters that Globalisation can be Wished Away. *The Economist*, 15th November. www. economist.com/news/united-states/21632599-politicians-need-stop-pretending-angry-voters-globalisation-can-be-wished. [accessed 31st July, 2015)

Library and Archives Canada (1994) Persons Sentenced to Death in Canada, 1867–1976: Ka-ki-si-kutchin (alias Swift Runner) Government Archives Division1994 – An Inventory of Case Files. Ottawa, Ontario: National Archives of Canada.

Lichtenstein, P., Yip, B., Björk, C., Pawitan, Y., Cannon, T., Sullivan, P., and Hultman, C. (2009) Common Genetic Determinants of Schizophrenia and Bipolar Disorder in Swedish Families: A Population-Based Study. *Lancet*, 373(9659), pp. 234–239.

Liddle, R. (2009) It is the Narcissistic Middle-aged, Not the Young, Who Love Facebook and Twitter. *Spectator*, 15th July.

Liddle, R. (2014) *Selfish Whining Monkeys: How we Ended Up Greedy, Narcissistic and Unhappy*. London: Fourth Estate.

Lieberman, J. (2015) *Shrinks: The Untold Story of Psychiatry*. London: Weidenfeld & Nicolson.

Lindberg, C. (1992) *The Beginnings of Western Science: The European Scientific Tradition in Philosophical, Religious, and Institutional Context, 600 B.C. to A.D. 1450*. Chicago, IL: University of Chicago.

Linklater, A. (2013) *Why Spencer Perceval Had to Die: The Assassination of a British Prime Minister*. London: Bloomsbury.

Lipman, F. (2009) *Spent: End Exhaustion & Feel Great Again*. London: Hay House.

Littlewood, R. (2002) *Pathologies of the West*. London: Continuum.

Lodhi, A., and Tilly, C. (1973) Urbanization, Crime and Collective Violence in 19th century France. *American Journal of Sociology*, 79(2), pp. 296–318.

Lotringer, E. (1996) (editor) I, Pierre Rivière ... An Interview with Michel Foucault (1976) *Foucault Live: Collected Interviews, 1961–1984*, pp. 203–206. New York: Semiotext(e).

Lovelock, J. (2010) *The Vanishing Face of Gaia: A Final Warning*. London: Penguin.

Lukes, S. (2004) (second edition) *Power: A Radical View*. Basingstoke; Palgrave Macmillan.

MaCrae F (2013) The Lost Souls of 'Bedlam' Are Found. *Daily Mail*, 8th August.

McCulloch, J. (2006) *Colonial Psychiatry and the African Mind*. Cambridge: Cambridge University Press.

McCulloch, A., Muijen, M., and Harper, H. (2000) New Developments in Mental Health Policy in the United Kingdom. *International Journal of Law and Psychiatry*, 23(3–4), pp. 261–276.

McGinty, S. (2012) The Two Sides of RD Laing. *The Scotsman*, 13th October. www. scotsman.com/news/stephen-mcginty-the-two-sides-of-rd-laing-1-2573369. [accessed 10th April, 2014].

MacKenzie, P. (2014) Psychopathy, Antisocial Personality & Sociopathy: The Basics A History Review. *The Forensic Examiner*. www.theforensicexaminer.com/2014/pdf/MacKenzie_714.pdf. [accessed 20th October, 2015].

McLaren, N. (2007) *Humanizing Madness: Psychiatry and the Cognitive Neuroscience*. Ann Arbor, MI: Future Psychiatry.

McLeod, K. (1862) Two Cases Illustrative of Two Distinct Forms of Mania, with General Paralysis. *Journal of Mental Science* [which became the *British Journal of Psychiatry*], 7(40), pp. 546–559.

Main, T. (1946) The Hospital as a Therapeutic Institution. *Bulletin of the Menninger Clinic*, 10, pp. 66–70.

Makhlouf, F., and Rambaud, C. (2014) Child Homicide and Neglect in France: 1991–2008. *Child Abuse and Neglect*, January, 38(1), pp. 37–41.

Malik, K. (1998) The Darwinian Fallacy. *Prospect Magazine*, 20th December, www.prospectmagazine.co.uk/features/thedarwinianfallacy. [accessed 26th January, 2016].

Marano, L. (1982) Windigo Psychosis: The Anatomy of an Emic-Etic Confusion. *Current Anthropology*, 23, 385–412.

Marston, H. (2013) Information for the Public: A Brief History of Psychiatric Drug Development. *The British Association for Psychopharmachology*. 18th May. www.bap.org.uk/publicinformationitem.php?publicinfoID=24 [accessed 18th November, 2015].

Martin, J. (2002) The Integration of Neurology, Psychiatry, and Neuroscience in the 21st Century. *The American Journal of Psychiatry*, 159(5), pp. 695–704.

Marx, K. (1932) (written in 1844) *Economic and Philosophic Manuscripts of 1844* [translated by Mulligan, M.]. Moscow: Progress.

Marx, K. (1852) *The Eighteenth Brumaire of Louis Napoleon* [*Der 18te Brumaire des Louis Napoleon*]. Die Revolution, 1. www.marxists.org/archive/marx/works/1852/18th-brumaire/ch01.htm [accessed 2nd May, 2015].

Marx, K. (1867; 1885; 1894) *Das Kapital, Kritik der Politischen Ökonomie* [*Capital: Critique of Political Economy*; volumes I, II, and III]. Hamburg: Meissner.

Mason, R. (2013) David Cameron Met Stephen Fry to Discuss Russian Gay Rights Row. *The Guardian*, 18th August.

Measham, F., and Brain, K. (2005) 'Binge' Drinking, British Alcohol Policy and the New Culture of Intoxication. *Crime Media Culture*, 1(3), pp. 262–283.

Megget, K. (2016) Crispr Goes Commercial. *ChemistryWorld* [Royal Society of Chemistry]. www.chemistryworld.com/business/crispr-goes-commercial/9359.article. [accessed 26th August, 2016].

Melle, I. (2013) The Breivik Case and what Psychiatrists can Learn from it. *World Psychiatry*, 12(1), pp. 16–21.

Mellett, D. (1982) *The Prerogative of Asylumdom: Social, Cultural and Administrative Aspects of the Institutional Treatment of the Insane in Nineteenth-Century Britain*. New York: Taylor and Francis.

Melling, J., and Forsyth, B. (1999) (editors) *Insanity, Institutions and Society, 1800–1914: A Social History of Madness in Comparative Perspective*. London, Routledge.

Mental Health Act 2007 (2007), Part 1 Amendments to Mental Health Act 1983. London: Department of Health.

Mental Health Foundation (2013) *Starting Today: Future of Mental Health Services. Final Inquiry Report*. London: Mental Health Foundation.

Mental Health Tribunal (2013) First-tier Tribunal (Health, Education and Social Care) (Mental Health) and in the Matter of an Application by Ian Stuart Brady. www.judiciary.gov.uk/wp-content/uploads/JCO/Documents/Judgments/ian-brady-mh-tribunal-240114.pdf. [accessed 14th February, 2015].

Merton, R. (1938) Social Structure and Anomie. *American Sociological Review*, 3 (October), pp. 672–682.

Merton, R. (1949) *Social Theory and Social Structure*. New York: Free Press.

Merton, R. (1957) *Social Theory and Social Structure*. New York: Free Press.

Midgley, M. (1994) *Science as Salvation: A Modern Myth and its Meaning*. London: Routledge.

Miko, I. (2008) Gregor Mendel and the Principles of Inheritance. *Nature Education*, 1(1), p.134.

Miller, G. (2004) *R D Laing*. Edinburgh: Edinburgh Review/Edinburgh University Press.

Miller, J. (1993) *The Passion of Michel Foucault*. New York: Simon & Schuster.

Miller, P., and Rose, N. (1986) (editors) *The Power of Psychiatry*. London: Blackwell/Polity.

Mills, C. (2014) *Decolonising Global Mental Health: The Psychiatrization of the Majority World*. New York: Routledge.

Mills, C. W. (1956) *The Power Elite*. Oxford: Oxford University Press.

Mills, S. (2003) *Michel Foucault*. London: Routledge.

Mind For Therapy (2016) R. D. Laing's Connection to Family Therapy. www.mindfortherapy.com/laing-and-family-therapy.html. [accessed 5th January, 2016].

Monbiot, G. (2007) *Heat: How We Can Stop the Planet Burning*. London: Penguin.

Moncrieff, J. (2009) *The Myth of the Chemical Cure: A Critique of Psychiatric Drug Treatment*. Basingstoke: Palgrave Macmillan

Moncrieff, J., and Feltham, C. (2013) The Interview: The Meaning of Madness. *Therapy Today*, 25(5). www.therapytoday.net/article/show/3762/the-interview-the-meaning-in-madness/. [accessed 20th April, 2015].

Monk, L (2009) Working in the Asylum: Attendants to the Insane. *Health and History*, 11(1), 83–101.

Moore, D. (2015). *The Developing Genome: An Introduction to Behavioral Epigenetics*. Oxford: Oxford University Press.

Mora, G. (1972) On the Bicentenary of the Birth of Esquirol (1772–1840), the First Complete Psychiatrist. *American Journal of Psychiatry*, 129 (November), pp. 562–567.

Morrall, P. (1998) *Mental Health Nursing and Social Conrol*. London: Whurr.

Morrall, P. (2000) *Madness and Murder*. London: Whurr.

Morrall, P. (2008) *The Trouble With Therapy: Sociology and Psychotherapy*. Chichester: Open University Press/McGraw-Hill.

Morrall, P. (2009) (second edition) *Sociology and Health*. London: Routledge.

Morrall, P. (2016) Madness – Fear and Fascination. In: Chadee D (editor) *Psychology of Fear, Crime and the Media: International Persepctive*. New York: Routledge. Chapter 3, pp. 40–57.

Morrall, P., and Hazelton, M. (2000) Architecture Signifying Social Control: The Restoration of Asylumdom in Mental Health Care? *Australian and New Zealand Journal of Mental Health Nursing*, 9(2), pp. 89–96.

Morrall, P., and Hazelton, M. (2004) *Mental Health: Global Policies and Human Rights*. Chichester: Wiley.

Morrall, P., and Muir-Cochrane, E. (2002) Naked Social Control: Seclusion and Psychiatric Nursing in Post-Liberal Society. *Australian e-Journal for the Advancement of Mental Health*, 1(2), pp. 101–112.

Mosely, I. (2000) (editor) *Dumbing Down: Culture, Politics and the Mass Media*. Exeter; Imprint Academic.

Morrison, L. (2013) *Talking Back To Psychiatry: The Psychiatric Consumer/Survivor/Ex-Patient Movement*. New York: Routledge.

Moustakas, C. (1994) *Phenomenological Research Methods*. London: Sage.

Mukherjee, S. (2016) *The Gene: An Intimate History*. London: Bodley Head.

Mullan, B. (1999) *R.D. Laing: A Personal View*. London: Duckworth.

Mullan, R. (2017) (writer/director) *Mad to be Normal* [film]. London: Gizmo Films, GSP Studios & Bad Penny Productions

Narayan, C., and Shikha, D. (2013) Indian Legal System and Mental Health. *Indian Journal of Psychiatry*, 55(Suppl 2), pp. 177–181.

Nasrallah, H. (2011) The Antipsychiatry Movement: Who and Why. *Current Psychiatry*, 10(12). www.currentpsychiatry.com/index.php?id=22661&tx_ttnews%5Btt_news%5D=176468. [accessed 6th January, 2016].

National Aeronautics and Space Administration (2014) Taking a Global Perspective on Earth's Climate. Houston, TX: NASA. http://climate.nasa.gov/nasa_role. [accessed 22nd June, 2014].

National Institute for Health and Care Excellence (2014) Clinical Knowledge Summaries. http://cks.nice.org.uk/syphilis [accessed 18th March, 2016].

National Institute for Health and Care Excellence (2015) NICE Guidance on Helping NHS Staff to Deal with Violence and Aggression from Patients. www.nice.org.uk/news/press-and-media/nice-guidance-on-helping-nhs-staff-to-deal-with-violence-and-aggression-from-patients. [accessed 4th November, 2015].

National Institutes (USA) of Health (2013) Common Genetic Factors Found in Five Mental Disorders. www.nih.gov/researchmatters/march2013/03182013mental.htm. [accessed 20th April, 2015].

National Library of Medicine [USA] (2015). Mental Disorders. www.nlm.nih.gov/medlineplus/mentaldisorders.htm [accessed 25th January, 2016].

National Public Radio (2005). USA National Public Radio 'My Lobotomy': Howard Dully's Journey. www.npr.org/2005/11/16/5014080/my-lobotomy-howard-dullys-journey. [accessed 3rd November, 2015].

Nicol, W. D. (1956) General Paralysis of the Insane. *British Journal of Venereal Diseases*, 32(1), pp. 9–16.

Nietzsche, F. (1886) *Beyond Good and Evil: Prelude to a Philosophy of the Future* [*Jenseits von Gut und Böse: Vorspiel einer Philosophie der Zukunft*]. Leipzig: Naumann.

Nissim, M. (2012) Showbiz News: Stephen Fry is the Celebrity that Most Brits Would Want as PM. Digital Spy. www.digitalspy.co.uk/showbiz/news/a359716/stephen-fry-is-the-celebrity-that-most-brits-would-want-as-pm.html#~oMgwDYNpqSNeOK. [accessed 2nd May 2015].

Nolan, P. (1993) *A History of Mental Health Nursing*. London: Chapman and Hall.

Nsereko, D. (2011) *Criminal Law in Botswana*. Alphen aan den Rijn: Wolter Kluwer.

Oakes, J. (2006) Oedipal Issues in Shakespeare's *Antony and Cleopatra*, Ibsen's *Hedda Gabler* and Foucault's *I, Pierre Rivière, Having Slaughtered my Mother, my Sister and my Brother…* http://motif.janetoakes.com/1/post/2011/12/oedipal-issues.html. [accessed 20th April, 2014].

O'Brien, T. (2005) *Mary Barnes* by Mary Barnes and Joseph Berkes. *Metapsychology: Book Reviews*, 9(8). http://metapsychology.mentalhelp.net/poc/view_doc.php?type=book&id=2552&cn=392. [accessed 29th February, 2016].

O'Hagan, S. (2012) Kingsley Hall: RD Laing's Experiment in Anti-psychiatry. *The Observer*, 2nd September.

Onions, C. (1966) *Oxford Dictionary of English Etymology*. Oxford: Oxford University Press.

van-Os, J. and Kapur, S. (2009) Schizophrenia. *The Lancet*, 374, 9690, pp. 635–645.

Otterson, J. (2014) *The End of Socialism*. Cambridge: Cambridge University Press.

Owen, J. (2006) Stephen Fry: My Battle with Mental Illness. *The Independent Sunday*, 17th September.

Oxfam (2014) Working For the Few: Political Capture and Economic Inequality [briefing paper 178]. Oxford: Oxfam.

Parker, S. (1960) The Wiitiko Psychosis in the Context of Ojibwa Personality and Culture. *American Anthropologist*, 62(4), pp. 602–655.

Paterson, T., and Taylor, J. (2011) What Turned Anders Breivik into Norway's Worst Nightmare? *The Independent*, 28th July.

Patton, M. (2015) RD Laing: Was the Counterculture's Favourite Psychiatrist a Dangerous Renegade or a True Visionary? *The Independent*, 30th November.

Pearce, J. (2004) The Argyll Robertson Pupil. *Neurology, Neurosurgery, and Psychiatry*, 75(9), p. 1345.

Perceval, J .(1840) *A Narrative of the Treatment Experienced by a Gentleman during a State of Mental Derangement; Designed to Explain the Causes and the Nature of Insanity, and to Expose the Injudicious Conduct Pursued Towards Many Unfortunate Sufferers under that Calamity by John Perceval Esq.* London: Effingham Wilson, Royal Exchange.

Peterson, A., and Bunton, R. (2012) *Foucault, Health and Medicine*. London: Routledge.

Peterson, D. (1982) (editor) *A Mad People's History of Madness*. Pittsburgh, PA: University of Pittsburgh.

Pies, R. (2013) Context Does Not Determine 'Disorderness' or Normality. *Psychiatric Times*, 15th January, pp. 1–2. www.psychiatrictimes.com/articles/context-does-not-determine-%E2%80%9Cdisorderness%E2%80%9D-or-normality. [accessed 1st August, 2014].

Pinker, S. (2012) *The Better Angels of Our Nature: A History of Violence and Humanity*. London: Penguin.

Pinker, S. (2013) Science Is not your Enemy: An Impassioned Plea to Neglected Novelists, Embattled Professors, and Tenure-Less Historians. *New Republic*, 7th August. https://newrepublic.com/article/114127/science-not-enemy-humanities. [accessed 2nd March, 2016].

PinkNews (2011) Stephen Fry says he Finds Fame 'Exhausting' and that Suicide is Always an Option. 2nd June. www.pinknews.co.uk/2011/06/02/stephen-fry-says-he-finds-fame-exhausting-and-that-suicide-is-always-an-option/. [accessed 2nd May, 2015].

Pippard, J., and Ellam, L. (1981). Electroconvulsive Treatment in Great Britain. *British Journal of Psychiatry*, 139(6), pp. 563–568.

Pope Francis (2014) Quoted in: Kaufman, A. (2014) Pope Francis Warns the Global Economy is near Collapse. *Huffington Post*, www.huffingtonpost.com/2014/06/13/pope-francis-economy_n_5491831.html. [accessed 29th January, 2016].

Popper, K .(1959) *The Logic of Scientific Discovery*. New York: Harper and Row.

Porter, R. (1987) *A Social History of Madness: Stories of the Insane*. London: Weidenfeld & Nicolson.

Porter, R. (2002) *Blood and Guts: A Short History of Medicine*. London: Penguin.

Porter, R. (2003) *Madness: A Brief History*. Oxford: Oxford University Press.

Powledge, T. (2014) Does the Human 'Warrior Gene' make Violent Criminals – And what should Society Do? *Genetic Literacy Project*, 4th November. http://geneticliteracyproject.org/2014/11/04/does-the-human-warrior-gene-make-violent-criminals-and-what-should-society-do/ [accessed 29th January, 2016].

Priebe, S. (2015) The Political Mission of Psychiatry. *World Psychiatry: Official Journal of the World Psychiatric Association*, 14(1), pp. 1–2.

Proceedings of the Old Bailey (1812) John Bellingham, Killing – Murder, 13th May 1812. www.oldbaileyonline.org/browse.jsp?id=t18120513-5&div=t18120513-5. [accessed 30th October, 2015].

Psychiatric Genomics Consortium (2014) Biological Insights From 108 Schizophrenia -associated Genetic Loci. [Schizophrenia Working Group]. *Nature*, 511(7510), pp. 421–427.

Psychiatric Genomics Consortium (2015) Psychiatric Genome-wide Association Study Analyses Implicate Neuronal, Immune and Histone Pathways [The Network and Pathway Analysis Subgroup]. *Nature Neuroscience*, 18(2), pp. 199–209.

Purcell, S., Wray, N., Stone, J., Visscher, P., O'Donovan, M., Sullivan, P. and Sklar, P. (2009) Common Polygenic Variation Contributes to Risk of Schizophrenia and Bipolar Disorder. *Nature* 460, 748–752.

Radkau, J. (2011) *Max Weber: A Biography*. Cambridge: Polity.

Rafferty, A., Webster, C., and Dingwall, R. (1988) *An Introduction to the Social History of Nursing*. London: Routledge.

Ralley, O. (2012) *The Rise of Anti-psychiatry: A Historical Review*. www.priory.com/history_of_medicine/Anti-Psychiatry.htm. [accessed 12th January, 2016].

Ramakrishnan, V. (2016) More Than Ever, Science Must be Central to All Our Lives. *The Observer*, 28th February.

Rawnsley A (2016) Terrifying Trump will turn into Tamed Trump? It's an illusion. *The Observer*, 13th November.

Read, J., and Dillon, J. (2013) (second edition) (editors) *Models of Madness: Psychological, Social and Biological Approaches to Psychosis*. London: Routledge.

Reiss, J., and Sprenger, J. (2014) *Scientific Objectivity: Stanford Encyclopedia of Philosophy*. Stanford, CA: Stanford University. http://plato.stanford.edu/entries/scientific-objectivity/. [accessed 22nd August, 2015].

Reuters Canada (2015) Breivik Bomb Van Exhibited on Norway Massacre Anniversary. 15th July. http://ca.reuters.com/article/topNews/idCAKCN0PP1KW20150715. [accessed 23rd October, 2015].

Richard Dawkins Foundation (2016) Genetic Study Provides First-Ever Insight into Biological Origin of Schizophrenia. https://richarddawkins.net/2016/01/genetic-study-provides-first-ever-insight-into-biological-origin-of-schizophrenia/. [accessed 8th February, 2016].

Rissmiller, D., and Rissmiller, J. (2006) Open Forum: Evolution of the Antipsychiatry Movement Into Mental Health Consumerism. *Psychiatric Services*, 57, pp. 863–866.

Ritchie, S. (2016) On Genetics Oliver James is on a Different Planet to the Rest of Us. *The Spectator*, 8th March. http://health.spectator.co.uk/on-genetics-oliver-james-is-wrong-about-everything/. [accessed 15th March, 2016].

Rix, K. (2011) *Expert Psychiatric Evidence*. London: Royal College of Psychiatry.

Roberts, M. (2005) The Production of the Psychiatric Subject: Power, Knowledge and Michel Foucault. *Nursing Philosophy*, 6(1), pp. 33–42.

Robinson, P. (1972) (director) *Asylum* [film]. London: Peter Robinson Associates.

Robinson, D., and Williams, R. (2015) (editors) *Scientism: The New Orthodoxy*. London: Bloomsbury.

Rogers, A., and Pilgrim, D. (2003) *Mental Health and Inequality*. Basingstoke: Palgrave.

Rogers, A., and Pilgrim, D. (2014) (fifth edition) *A Sociology of Mental Health and Illness*. Maidenhead: Open University-Press/McGraw-Hill.

Ronson, J. (2012) (new edition) *The Psychopath Test*. London: Picador.

Rose, H., and Rose, S. (2001) *Alas Poor Darwin: Arguments Against Evolutionary Psychology*. London: Vintage.

Rose, N. (1998) Controversies in Meme Theory. *Journal of Memetics – Evolutionary Models of Information Transmission*, 2. http://cfpm.org/jom-emit/1998/vol2/rose_n.html. [accessed 21st April, 2015].

Rose, N. (2006) *The Politics of Life Itself: Biomedicine, Power, and Subjectivity in the Twenty-First Century*. Princeton, NJ: Princeton University Press.

Rose, N. (2010) Screen and Intervene: Governing Risky Brains. *[Journal of] History of the Human Sciences: Special Issue on the New Brain Sciences*, 23(1), pp. 79–105.

Rose, N. (2013) The Human Sciences in a Biological Age. *Theory, Culture and Society*, 30(1), pp. 3–34.

Rose, N. (2016) Books and Articles. http://nikolasrose.com/. [accessed 16th March, 2016].

Rose, N., and Abi-Rached, J. (2013) *Neuro: The New Brain Sciences and the Management of the Mind*. Princeton, NJ: Princeton University Press.

Rose, S., and McGuffin, P. (2005) Will Science Explain Mental Illness?. *Prospect Magazine*, October, pp. 28–32.

Rosenberg, J. (2014) Mass Shootings and Mental Health Policy. *Journal of Sociology and Social Welfare*, 41(1), pp. 107–121.

Rosenhan, D. L. (1973) On Being Sane In Insane Places. *Science*, 179, pp. 250–258.

Rössler, W. and Meise, U. (1994) Wilhelm Griesinger and the Concept of Community Care in 19th-Century Germany. *Hospital and Community Psychiatry – American Psychiatric Association*, 45 (August), pp. 818–822.

Rowe, J. (2004) Brislington – An Historical View. www.brislington.org/history.html [accessed 3rd August, 2013].

Royal College of Psychiatrists (2013) Timeline of Psychiatry/History of Psychiatry. www.rcpsych.ac.uk/discoverpsychiatry/studentassociates/psychiatryinthemedia/historyofpsychiatry.aspx. [accessed 30th March, 2015].

Royal College of Psychiatrists (2015) Schizophrenia. www.rcpsych.ac.uk/healthadvice/problemsdisorders/schizophrenia.aspx [accessed 1st October, 2015].

Royal College of Psychiatrists (2016) Medications for Bipolar Disorder. www.rcpsych.ac.uk/healthadvice/treatmentswellbeing/medicationsbipolardisorder.aspx.[accessed 25th January, 2016].

Royal Society of Medicine (2005) Psychiatry and Society: Will neuroscience Change Understandings and Practices? www.rsm.ac.uk/events/events-listing/2014-2015/sections/psychiatry-section/pyf04-psychiatry-and-society-will-neuroscience-change-understandings-and-practices.aspx. [accessed 23rd March, 2006].

Ruscio, J. (2004) Diagnoses and the Behaviors They Denote: A Critical Evaluation of the Labeling Theory of Mental Illness. *The Scientific Review of Mental Health Practice*, 3(1). www.srmhp.org/0301/labels.html. [accessed 5th August, 2015].

Russell, B. (1961) *History of Western Civilisation*. London: Routledge.

Russell, D. (1995) *Women, Madness & Medicine*. Cambridge: Polity.

Rutherford, S. (2008) *The Victorian Asylum*. London: Colchester: Shire.

Saindon, J. (1933) Mental Disorders Among the James Bay Cree. *Primitive Man* [Quarterly Bulletin of the Catholic Anthropological Conference], 6(1), pp. 1–12.

Sample, I. (2015) New Study Claims to Find Genetic Link Between Creativity and Mental Illness. *The Guardian*, 8th June.

Sartre, J. (1965) (first published 1938) *Nausea [La Nausée]*. Harmondsworth, London: Penguin.

Schaler, J. (2012) Thomas Stephen Szasz: April 15, 1920 – September 8, 2012. www.szasz.com/szaszdeath.htm. [accessed 12th January, 2016].

Scheff, T. (1966) *Being Mentally Ill: A Sociological Theory*. Chicago: Aldine.

Schlesinger, J. (2012) *The Insanity Hoax*. New: York: Shrinktunes Media.

Schwartz, M. (2010) The Emergence of a New Science of the Mind: Immunology Benefits the Mind. *Molecular Psychiatry*, 15, pp. 337–338.

Science Council (2016) Our Definition of Science. http://sciencecouncil.org/about-us/our-definition-of-science. [accessed 2nd March 2016].

Scott, S. (2014) Psychopathy – An Evolving and Controversial Construct. *Psychiatry, Psychology and Law*, 21(5), pp. 687–715.

Scott, S., and Thorpe, C. (2006) The Sociological Imagination of R. D. Laing. *Sociological Theory*, 24(4), pp. 331–352.

Scull, A. (1977) *Decarceration: Community Treatment and the Deviant – A Radical View*. New York: Prentice-Hall.

Scull, A. (1979) *Museums of Madness: The Social Organisation of Insanity in Nineteenth-Century England*. London: Allen Lane.

Scull, A. (1984) (second edition) *Decarceration: Community Treatment and the Deviant – a Radical View*. Cambridge: Polity Press.

Scull, A. (1992) *Social Order – Mental Disorder: Anglo-American Psychiatry in Historical Perspective*. Berkeley, CA: University of California Press.

Scull, A. (1993a) *The Most Solitary of Afflictions. Madness and Society in Britain 1700–1900*, New Haven, CT: Yale University.

Scull, A. (1993b) Museums of Madness Revisited. *Social History of Medicine* 6(1), pp. 3–23.

Scull, A. (2005a) 'Killing Cures': An Exchange. *The New York Review of Books*, 3rd November. www.nybooks.com/articles/archives/2005/nov/03/killing-cures-an-exchange/ [accessed 6th March, 2015].

Scull, A. (2005b) *Madhouse: A Tragic Tale of Megalomania and Modern Medicine*. London: Yale University Press.

Scull, A. (2007a) Scholarship of Fools. The Frail Foundations of Foucault's Monument. *The Times Literary Supplement*, 23rd March, pp. 3–4.

Scull, A. (2007b) Mind, Brain, Law and Culture – Book reviews by Andrew Scull. *Brain*, 130, pp. 585–591.

Scull, A. (2010) A Psychiatric Revolution. *The Lancet*, 375 (9722), pp. 1246–1247.

Scull, A. (2011) *Madness: A Very Short Introduction*. Oxford: Oxford University Press.

Scull, A. (2015) *Madness in Civilisation: From the Bible to Freud, from the Madhouse to Modern Medicine*. London: Thames & Hudson.

Seierstad, A. (2015) *One of Us: The Story of Anders Breivik and the Massacre in Norway*. London: Virago.

Sekar, A., Bialas, A., de Rivera, H., Davis, A., Hammond, T., Kamitaki, N., Tooley, K., Presumey, J., Baum, M., Van Doren, V., Genovese, G., Rose, S. A., Handsaker, R., Schizophrenia Working Group of the Psychiatric Genomics Consortium, Daly, M., Carroll, M., Stevens, B., and McCarroll, S. (2016). Schizophrenia Risk from Complex Variation of Complement Component 4, *Nature*, 530(7589), pp. 177-83.

Semple, D., and Smyth, R. (2013) *Oxford Handbook of Psychiatry*. Oxford: Oxford University Press.

Sheid, T., and Brown, T. (2011) (Second edition) *A Handbook for the Study of Mental Health: Social Contexts, Theories, and Systems*. Cambridge: Cambridge University Press.

Sheldrake, R. (2012) *The Science Delusion*. London: Coronet.

Shermer, M. (2015) *Moral Arc: How Science and Reason Lead Humanity Toward Truth Justice, and Freedom*. New York: Henry Holt.

Shorter, E. (1997) *A History of Psychiatry: From the Era of the Asylum to the Age of Prozac A History of Psychiatry*. New York: Wiley.

Showalter, E. (1987) *The Female Malady: Women, Madness and English Culture, 1830–1980*. London: Virago.

Shulman, K. (2000) Clock-drawing: Is it the Ideal Cognitive Screening Test? *International Journal of Geriatric Psychiatry*, 15(6), pp. 548–561.

Singh, A. (2010) Stephen Fry is a National Treasure says Prince Charles. *The Telegraph*, 21st January.

Smith, J. (2009) *Interpretative Phenomenological Analysis: Theory, Method and Research*. London: Sage.

Smith, L. (1988) Behind Closed Doors; Lunatic Asylum Keepers, 1800–60. *Social History of Medicine* 1 (Dec. 1988).

Smith, L. (1999) *Cure, Comfort and Safe Custody: Public Lunatic Asylums in Early Nineteenth-Century England*. Leicester: Leicester University Press.

Smith, R., and Moynihan, R. (2002) Too Much Medicine? Almost Certainly. *British Medical Journal*, 13th April, 324, pp. 859–860.

Sneddon, R. (2008) *Technology in Times Past: Ancient Rome*. Mankato, MN: Black Rabbit.

Society for Cultural Anthropology (2015) SCA Prizes. www.culanth.org/pages/prizes#head. [accessed 13th November, 2015].

Society for Laingian Studies (2013) Bibliography: Politics and Other Works. http://laingsociety.org/biblio/books.htm. [accessed 16th February, 2014].

Sontag, S. (1989). *AIDS and Its Metaphors*. New York: Farrar-Straus-Giroux.

Sorell, T. (1994), *Scientism: Philosophy and the Infatuation with Science*. London: Routledge.

Spector, T. (2012) *Identically Different: Why You Can Change Your Genes*. London: Weidenfeld and Nicolson.

Sperling, D., and Gordon, D. (2009) *Two Billion Cars: Driving Toward Sustainability*. Oxford: Oxford University Press.

Sperry, L., and Sperry, J. (2015) *Cognitive Behavior Therapy of DSM-5 Personality Disorders: Assessment, Case Conceptualization, and Treatment*. London: Routledge.

Stephenfry.com (2016) Stephen Fry: The Old Friary. www.stephenfry.com/store/. [accessed 1st October, 2016].

Stern, A. (2005) Sterilized in the Name of Public Health, *American Journal of Public Health*, 95(7), pp. 1128–1138.

Stevens, A., and Price, J. (2000) (second edition) *Evolutionary Psychiatry: A New Beginning*. London: Routledge.

Stone, M. (1998) *Healing the Mind: A History of Psychiatry from Antiquity to the Present*. London: Pimlico.

Suibhne, S. (2011) Erving Goffman's Asylums 50 Years On. *The British Journal of Psychiatry*, 198, 1–2.

Smith L. (1988) Behind Closed Doors; Lunatic Asylum Keepers, 1800–60. *Social History of Medicine*, 1 (3), pp. 301–327.

Szasz, T. (1960) The Myth of Mental Illness. *American Psychologist*, 15, pp. 113–118.

Szasz, T. (1961) *The Myth of Mental Illness: Foundations of a Theory of Personal Conduct*. New York: Hoeber-Harper.

Szasz, T. (1970) *The Manufacture of Madness: A Comparative Study of the Inquisition and the Mental Health Movement*. New York: Harper and Row.

Szasz, T. (1976a) Anti-Psychiatry: The Paradigm of the Plundered Mind. *The New Review*, 3(29), pp. 3–14.

Szasz, T. (1976b) Schizophrenia: The Sacred Symbol of Psychiatry, *British Journal of Psychiatry*, 129(4), pp. 308–316.

Szasz, T. (1986) The Case Against Suicide Prevention. *American Psychologist*, 41(7), pp. 806–812.

Szasz, T. (1993) Curing, Coercing, and Claims-making: A Reply to Critics. *British Journal of Psychiatry*, 162(6), pp. 797–800.

Szasz, T. (1994) Mental Illness is Still a Myth. *Society*, 31(4), 34–39.

Szasz, T. (1998) Parity for Mental Illness, Disparity for the Mental Patient. *Lancet*, 352 (9135), 1213–1215.

Szasz, T. (2003) Psychiatry and the Control of Dangerousness: On the Apotropaic Function of the Term 'Mental Illness'. *Journal of Medical Ethics*, 29 (August), pp. 227–230.

Szasz, T. (2008). Debunking Antipsychiatry: Laing, Law, and Largactil. *Existential Analysis*, 19(2), 316–343.

Szasz, T. (2010a) The Illegitimacy of the 'Psychiatric Bible'. *The Freeman*, 60, pp. 16–18.

Szasz, T. (2010b) *Antipsychiatry: Quackery Squared*. New York: Syracuse University Press.

Taleb, N. (2006) *The Black Swan: The Impact of the Highly Improbable*. London: Palgrave Macmillan.

Tallis, R. (2004) (second edition) *Why the Mind is Not a Computer: A Pocket Lexicon of Neuromythology*. Exeter: Imprint Academic.

Tallis, R. (2014) *Aping Mankind: Neuromania, Darwinitis and the Misrepresentation of Humanity*. London: Routledge.

Tasman, A. (2014) The Most Exciting Time in the History of Psychiatry. *Psychiatric Times*, 15th October. www.psychiatrictimes.com/history-psychiatry/most-exciting-time-history-psychiatry. [accessed 3rd February, 2015].

Taylor, B. (2014) *The Last Asylum: A Memoir of Madness in Our Times*. London: Hamish Hamilton.

Taylor, C. B. (2012) *How to Practice Evidence-based Psychiatry: Basic Principes and Case Studies*. Washington DC: American Psychiatric Publishing.

Taylor, M. (2011) Psychopaths: Born Evil or with a Diseased Brain? BBC News, 15th November. www.bbc.co.uk/news/health-15386740. [accessed 19th April, 2014].

Theodossopoulos, D., and Kirtsoglo, E. (2010) *United in Discontent: Local Responses to Cosmopolitanism and Globalization*. Oxford: Berghahn.

Thomson, C. (1984) *Swift Runner*. Calgary: Detselig Enterprises.

Tiikkaja, S., Sandin, S., Malki, N., Modin, B., Sparén, P., and Hultman, C. (2013) Social Class, Social Mobility and Risk of Psychiatric Disorder – A Population-Based Longitudinal Study. *PLoS ONE* 15th November, 8(11). www.plosone.org/article/info:doi%2F10.1371%2Fjournal.pone.0077975. [accessed 6th May, 2015].

Time to Change (2008) Mind Your Language! www.time-to-change.org.uk/news-media/media-advisory-service/help-journalists/mind-your-language. [accessed 31st July, 2015].

Time To Change (2012) Stephen Fry Talks about Bipolar Disorder and Mental Health Stigma. www.time-to-change.org.uk/news-media/celebrity-supporters/stephen-fry. [accessed 26th January 2016].

Todorov, A., Fiske, A., and Prentice, D. (2014) (editors) *Social Neuroscience: Toward Understanding the Underpinnings of the Social Mind*. Oxford; Oxford University Press.

Trimble, R., and George, R. (2010) *Biological Psychiatry*. Chichester; Wiley-Blackwell.

Turner, C. (2015) Stephen Fry: Prince Charles Would Not 'Judge' me for Snorting Cocaine in Buckingham Palace. *The Telegraph*, 21st June.

Twenge, J. (2014) (revised edition) *Generation Me*. New York: Atria.

Twenge, J., and Campbell, W. (2009) *The Narcissism Epidemic: Living in the Age of Entitlement*. Free Press: New York.

Twitter (2016) Stephen Fry. https://twitter.com/stephenfry. [accessed 1st October, 2016].

United Nations (2015) Global Issues. www.un.org/en/globalissues/population/. [accessed 30th July 2015].

United Nations (2016) Global Issues: Refugees. www.un.org/en/globalissues/refugees/. [accessed 8th February, 2016].

United Nations Office on Drugs and Crime (2014) *Global Study on Homicide 2013: Trends, Contexts, Data*. Vienna: United Nations.

United Nations Population Fund (2015) Migration. www.unfpa.org/migration [accessed 8th February, 2016).

University of Liverpool (2015) Professor Richard Bentall [Staff Profiles]. www.liverpool. ac.uk/psychology-health-and-society/staff/richard-bentall/. [accessed 20th January, 2016].

Vanbergen G (2017) Global Discontent With Politics, Neoliberalism and Globalisation Rises. Centre for Research on Globalization, 26th. January www.globalresearch. ca/global-discontent-with-politics-neoliberalism-and-globalisation-rises/5570954. [accessed 13th February, 2017].

Vedral, V. (2010) *Decoding Reality: The Universe as Quantum Information*. Oxford: Oxford University Press.

Vernon, P. (2010) Stephen Fry Shocks Feminists by Claiming Women Don't Really Like Sex. *The Guardian*, 31st October.

Verona, E., and Patrick, C. (2015) Psychobiological Aspects of Antisocial Personality Disorder, Psychopathy, and Violence. *Psychiatric Times*. 25th March, 32(3). www. psychiatrictimes.com/special-reports/psychobiological-aspects-antisocial-personality-disorder-psychopathy-and-violence#sthash.9jmf7JlS.dpuf. [accessed 20th October, 2015].

Vickers, S. (2009) See a Psychiatrist? Are you Mad? *The Observer*, Sunday 21st June.

Wachtel, P., and Stanley, B. (1997) (editors) *Theories of Psychotherapy: Origins and Evolution*. Washington, DC: American Psychological Association.

Waldram, J. (James) (2004) *Revenge of the Windigo: The Construction of the Mind and Mental Health of North American Aboriginal Peoples*. Toronto: University of Toronto Press.

Walker, T. (2013) *The Events*, Young Vic, review. *The Telegraph*, 16th October. www.telegraph. co.uk/culture/theatre/theatre-reviews/10383346/The-Events-Young-Vic-review.html. [accessed 5th August, 2014].

Ward, E. (2010) Prostitution and the Irish State: From Prohibitionism to a Globalised Sex Trade. *Irish Political Studies*, 25(1), pp. 47–65.

Weber, M. (1947) *The Theory of Social and Economic Organization*. New York; Free Press.

Weber, M. (1978; original 1922) *Economy and Society [Wirtschaft und Gesellschaft]* Berkeley, CA: University of California Press.

Websdale, N. (2013) *Familicidal Hearts: The Emotional Styles of 211 Killers*. New York: Oxford University Press.

Weiner, D. (1992) Philippe Pinel's 'Memoir on Madness' of December 11, 1794: A Fundamental Text of Modern Psychiatry. *American Journal of Psychiatry*, June, 149(6), pp. 725–732.

Weiner, D. (1994) 'Le geste de Pinel: Psychiatric Myth,' in Micale M and Porter R (editors), *Discovering the History of Psychiatry*. Oxford, Oxford University Press, pp. 232–247.

Weir, K. (2012) The Roots of Mental Illness – How Much of Mental Illness can the Biology of the Brain Explain? *American Psychological Association*, 43(6), p.30. www.apa.org/pubs/ index.aspx.. [accessed 20th April, 2015].

Wessely, S., and James, O. (2013) Do We Need to Change the Way We Are Thinking about Mental Illness? *The Observer*, 12th May.

Western, D. (1998) The Scientific Legacy of Sigmund Freud: Toward a Psychodynamically Informed Psychological Science. *Psychological Bulletin*, 124(3), pp. 331–371.

Wexler, B. (2006) *Brain and Culture: Neurobiology, Ideology, and Social Change*. Cambridge, MA: Massachusetts Institute of Technology.

Whitaker, R. (2005) *Anatomy of an Epidemic: Magic Bullets, Psychiatric Drugs and the Astonishing Rise of Mental Illness in America*. New York: Crown Publishers.

Whitaker, R. (2010) (revised edition) *Mad in America: Bad Science, Bad Medicine, and the Enduring Mistreatment of the Mentally Ill*. New York: Basic Books.

Whitaker, R., and Cosgrave, L. (2015) *Psychiatry Under the Influence: Institutional Corruption, Social Injury, and Prescriptions for Reform*. London: Palgrave Macmillan.

White, D. (2013) *The Manipulation of Choice: Ethics and Libertarian Paternalism*. Basingstoke Palgrave Macmillan.

White, P. D., Rickards, H., and Zeman, A. (2012) Time to End the Distinction Between Mental and Neurological Illnesses. *British Medical Journal*, 344 [e3454]. www.bmj.com/content/344/bmj.e3454. [accessed 24th March, 2016].

Whitely, R. (2012) The Antipsychiatry Movement: Dead, Diminishing, or Developing? *Psychiatric Services*, 63(10), pp. 1039–1041.

Wiggershaus, R. (2010) *The Frankfurt School: Its History, Theory and Political Significance*. Cambridge: Polity.

Wilkinson, I. (2005) *Suffering: A Sociological Introduction*. Cambridge. Polity.

Wilkinson, R., and Pickett, K. (2010) *The Spirit Level: Why Equality is Better for Everyone*. London: Penguin.

William, P. (2012) *Rethinking Madness: Towards a Paradigm Shift in Our Understanding and Treatment of Psychosis*. San Francisco, CA: Sky's Edge.

Williams, R. (2011) How the Drug Companies are Controlling Our Lives Part 3: Evidence That Questions the Effectiveness Claims of Psychotropic Drugs. *Psychology Today*, 16th May. www.psychologytoday.com/blog/wired-success/201105/how-the-drug-companies-are-controlling-our-lives-part-3. [accessed 11th November, 2015].

Wilsdon, J., and Main, S. (2016) Anti-lobbying Clause Will Undermine Evidence, Policy and the Public Interest, says Chair. Campaign For Social Science. 18th February. https://campaignforsocialscience.org.uk/news/the-anti-lobbying-clause-will-undermine-evidence-policy-and-the-public-interest/. [accessed 21st February, 2016].

Wilson, E. O. (1975) *Sociobiology: The New Synthesis*. Cambridge, MA: Harvard University Press.

Wing, J. (1978) *Reasoning About Madness*. Oxford: Oxford University Press.

Wise, S. (2013) *Inconvenient People: Lunacy, Liberty and the Mad-Doctors in Victorian England*. London: Vintage.

Wolin, R. (2006) *The Frankfurt School Revisited*. London: Routledge.

Wolpert, L. (2000) (new edition) *The Unnatural Nature of Science*. London: Faber and Faber.

World Bank (2015) *Working for a World Free of Poverty*. www.worldbank.org/en/topic/poverty/overview. [accessed 28th July, 2015].

World Bank (2016) FAQs: Global Poverty Line Update. Washington DC: World Bank. www.worldbank.org/en/topic/poverty/brief/global-poverty-line-faq. [accessed 27th January, 2016].

World Health Organisation (2003) *Investing in Mental Health*. Geneva: World Health Organisation.

World Health Organisation (2005) *Improving Access and Use of Psychotropic Medicines*. Geneva: World Health Organisation.

World Health Organisation (2010) *International Statistical Classification of Diseases and Related Health Problems 10th Revision* (ICD-10) Version for 2010. Geneva: World Health Organisation. http://apps.who.int/classifications/icd10/browse/2010/en#/F60.8. [accessed 30th July, 2014].

World Health Organisation (2013) *Mental Health Action Plan 2013–2020*. Geneva: WHO.

World Health Organisation (2014a) *Mental Health: a State of Well-being* (Updated 14th August). www.who.int/features/factfiles/mental_health/en/. [accessed 30th January, 2015].

World Health Organisation (2014b) *Global Status Report on Violence Prevention 2014*. Geneva: World Health Organisation.

World Health Organisation (2015) *Gender and Women's Mental Health – Gender Disparities and Mental Health: The Facts.* www.who.int/mental_health/prevention/genderwomen/en/. [accessed 3rd May, 2015].

World Health Organisation (2016) *Schizophrenia.* www.who.int/mental_health/management/schizophrenia/en/. [accessed 8th January, 2016].

World Health Organisation/Gulbenkian Foundation (2014) *Social Determinants of Mental Health.* Geneva: World Health Organisation.

World Meteorological Organization (2016) Global Climate Breaks New Records January to June 2016. *World Meteorological Organization.* http://public.wmo.int/en/media/press-release/global-climate-breaks-new-records-january-june-2016. [accessed 14th September, 2016].

World Psychiatric Association (2015a) Transcultural Psychiatry: Introduction to its Field of Activity. *World Psychiatric Association* www.wpanet.org/detail.php?section_id=5&content_id=4. [accessed 29th April, 2015].

World Psychiatric Association (2015b) *Immunology and Psychiatry.* www.wpanet.org/detail.php?section_id=11&content_id=479. [accessed 24th August, 2016].

World Psychiatric Association (2016) *About the World Psychiatric Association: What are its Aims?* www.wpanet.org/detail.php?section_id=5&content_id=4 [accessed 2nd January, 2016].

Yang, H. (2011) Decoding the Biology of Bipolar Disorder: An Update on Recent Findings in Genetics, Imaging, and Immunology. *PsychiatryOnline* (Focus) 9, pp. 423–427. http://focus.psychiatryonline.org/article.aspx?articleid=181120. [accessed 27th July, 2014].

York, G. (1999) *The Dispossessed: Life and Death in Native Canada.* Toronto: McArthur.

Young-Bruehl, E. (1990) *Freud on Women.* London: Hogarth.

Zanor, C. (2010) A Fate That Narcissists Will Hate: Being Ignored. *New York Times*, 29th November. www.nytimes.com/2010/11/30/health/views/30mind.html. [accessed 9th November, 2014].

INDEX

Note: Page numbers followed by n indicate note numbers.

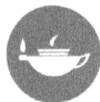